Nurse Dorothea® presents Anxiety and Managing It with Synergy

Authored by Michael Dow, RN, MS, MHA, MSM

Illustrations by Lindsay Roberts, M.Ed, BFA

Nurse Dorothea® presents
Anxiety and Managing It with Synergy

First Edition

ISBN 979-8-9905577-4-1

Printed by Lulu

Published by Dow Creative Enterprises®

Dow Creative Enterprises, LLC

PO Box 15357

Tucson, AZ 85708

Library of Congress Control Number: 2025908766

Dow Creative Enterprises® is a federally registered trademark with the United States Patent and Trademark Office.

Nurse Dorothea® is a federally registered trademark with the United States Patent and Trademark Office.

Help Civilization Reach Its Potential® is a federally registered trademark with the United States Patent and Trademark Office.

Table of Contents

Dedication

The Nurse Dorothea® book series is dedicated to Dorothea Dix. Her work in the 1800s helped people with mental illness live a more dignified life. She spent decades lobbying government officials to create state hospitals for the mentally ill. One person can make a difference.

Michael

Note to Reader

The Nurse Dorothea® book series is usually written in many parts. This book was an experiment to write more content on each page, so that it would be shorter, and the book would cost even less than a normal book in the series. I hope you enjoy this book as you have the others in the series.

Michael

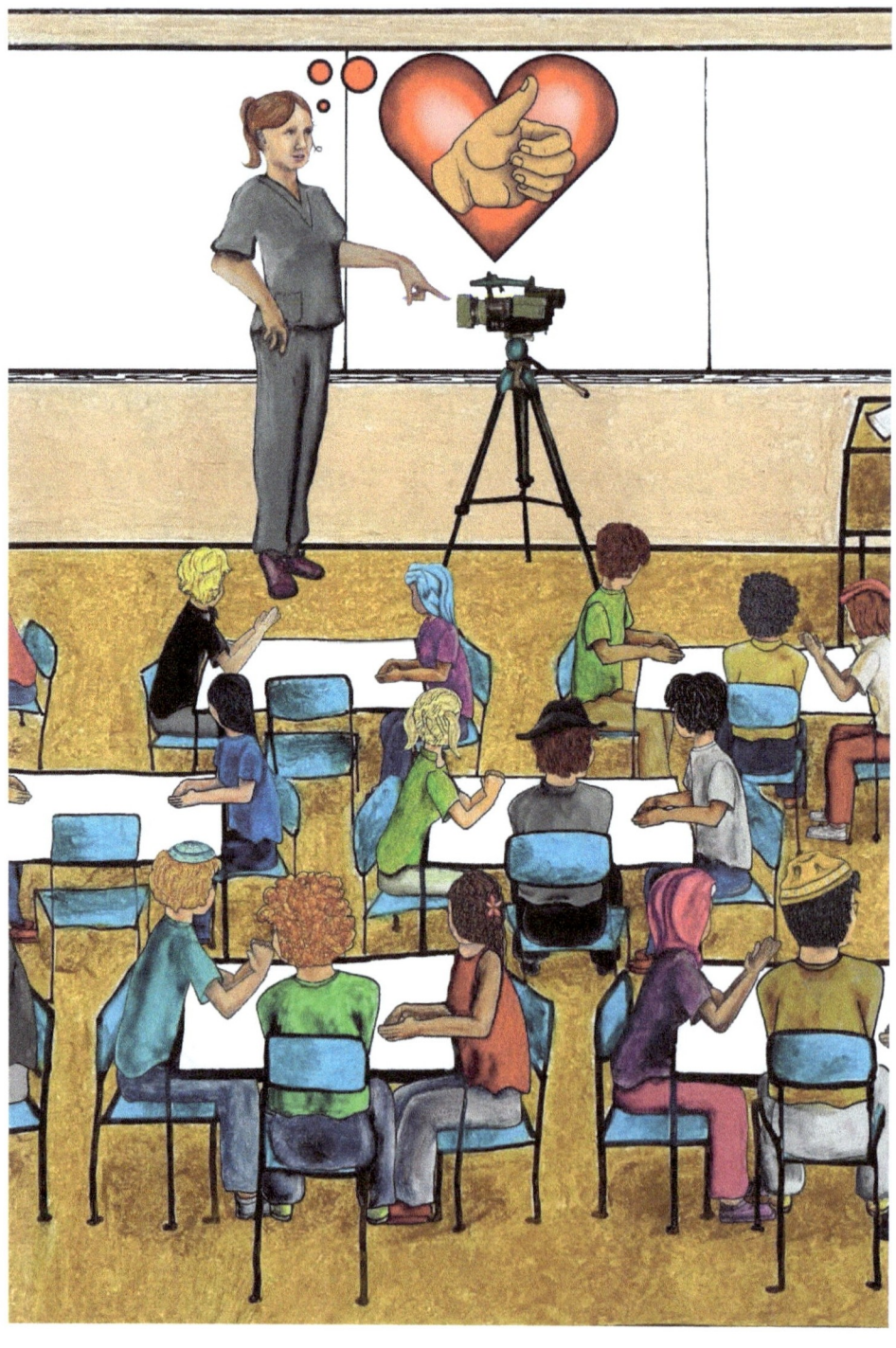

"Hi everyone. My name is Nurse Dorothea. Thank you for coming to the after-school club on mental health. I hope to provide you with some tools to manage your emotions and navigate life's challenges. Mental health is complicated because there are so many things that can affect it. This class was created to show that it's ok to talk about your mental health with others as well as give you ideas to improve your mental health. We will be recording this session. People in the future will get to experience the same things you will today. Sometimes, I will speak to people watching this show or reading the future book about the class. This is an interactive class, and I want you all to ask questions as you have them. We will stop sometimes and discuss things with each other. If you are watching the show or reading the book, then I want YOU all to also discuss the questions and topics with those in the room. This book is an experience, and you will only get the full experience by talking with others."

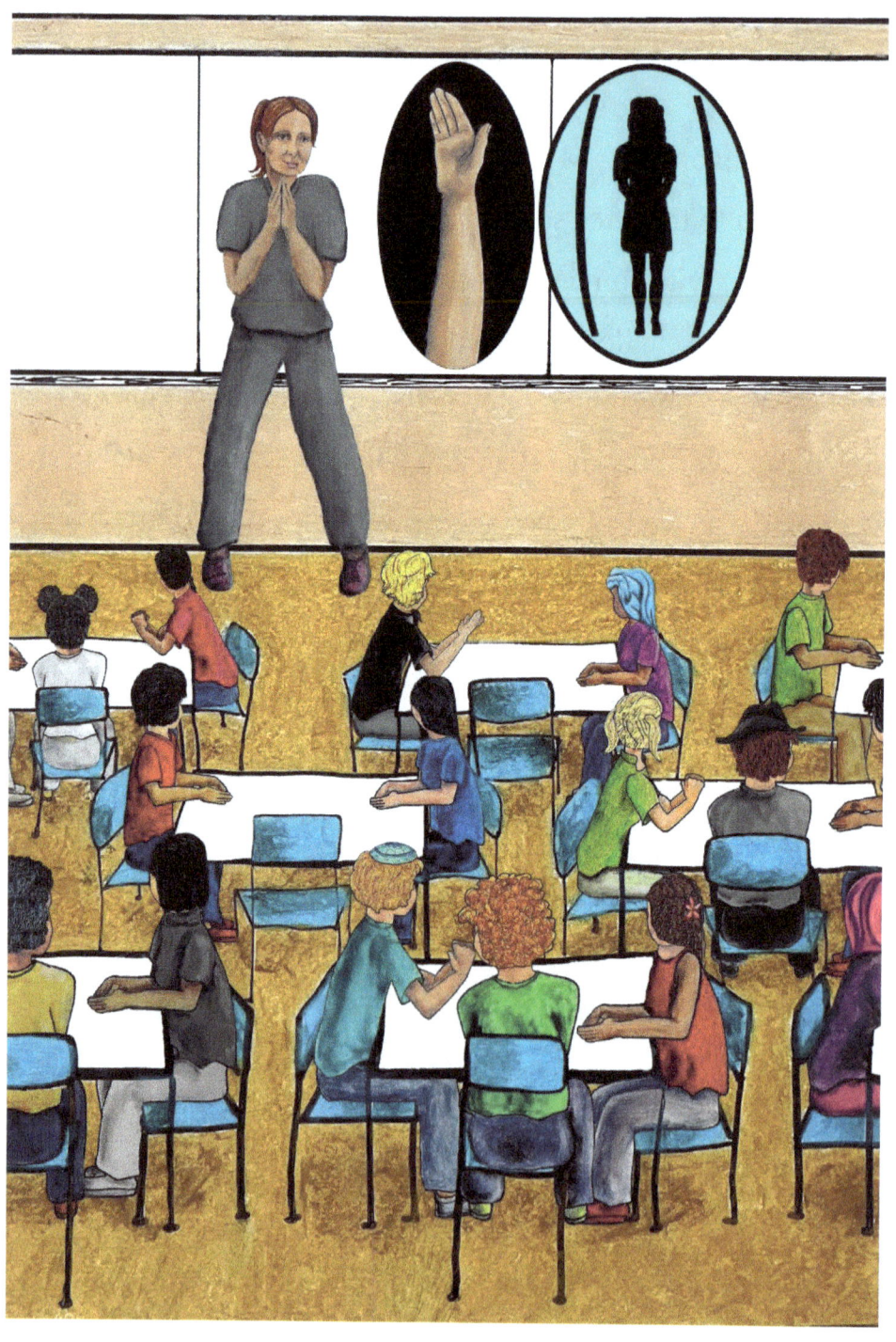

"If you are watching the show or reading this book alone, that is ok. Please take the time right now to get out a journal. I want those doing this class by themselves to write down responses to questions that I will ask, so that you participate like all the others. Sometimes, we need to address some mental health issues alone, so that is why it is ok to do this class by yourself. We are on a journey that is ultimately our own, but it is always nice to have people alongside us to help us in the bad times and share our joy in the good times. The main rule for the class is to respect others. If someone has a question, we are to be quiet and let them speak. Raise your hand if you have a question, and I will call on you. Respecting everyone is important since we can learn from everyone. To start the class, I'd like to mention that every person is one life event away from having a mental health challenge. Some people manage life events better than others, and one negative event for one person may cause depression and anxiety. For another person, it may only cause mild frustration because each person has different knowledge, skills, and abilities. This class is meant to help us have some common basic info."

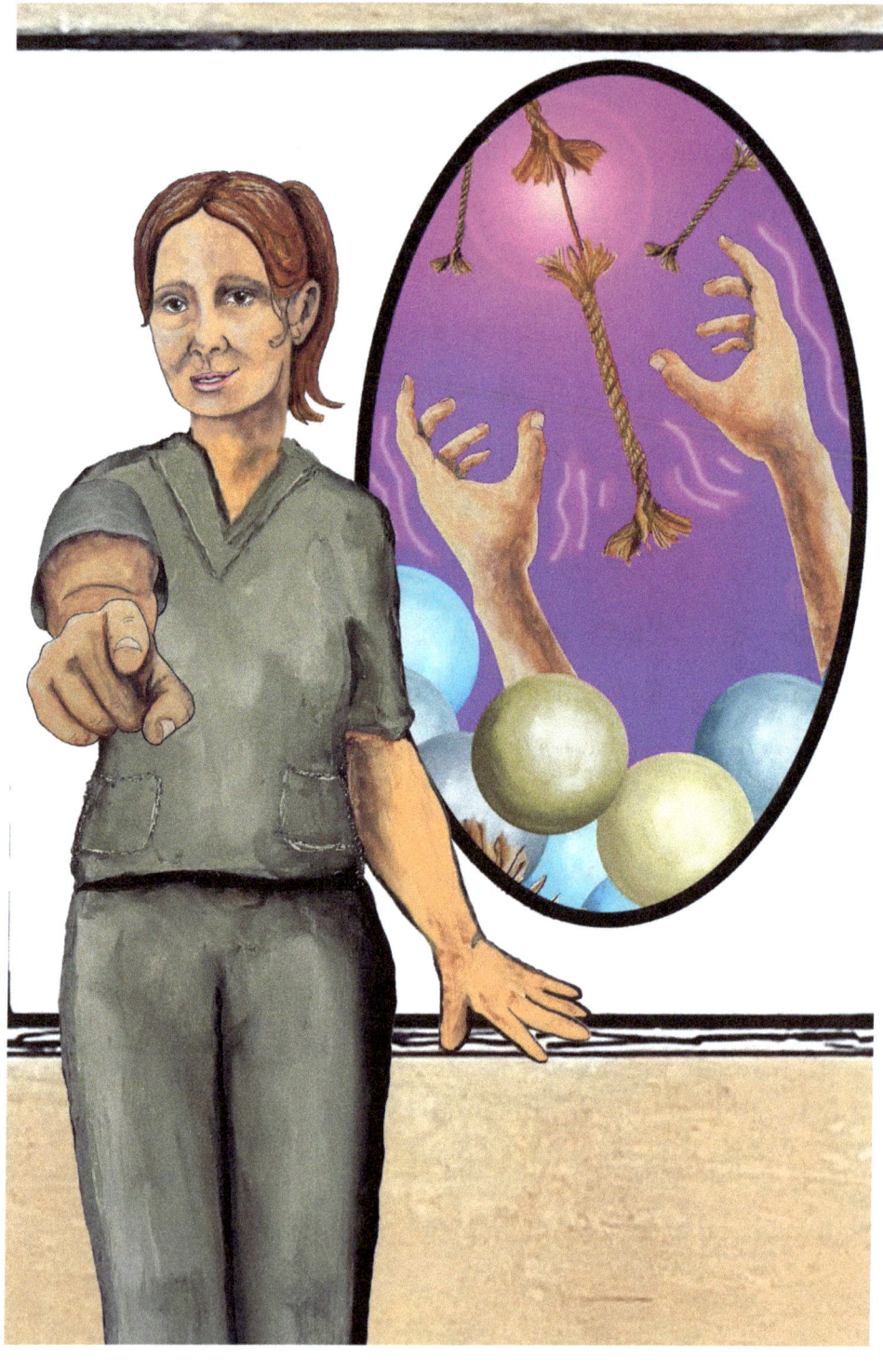

"This class will be about anxiety, which is a feeling we can experience in many different situations. Some experience it more strongly than others. *Merriam-Webster* defines anxiety as apprehensive uneasiness or nervousness usually over an impending or anticipated ill. The medical definition is an abnormal and overwhelming sense of apprehension and fear often marked by physical signs (such as tension, sweating, and increased pulse rate), by doubt concerning the reality and nature of the threat, and by self-doubt about one's capacity to cope with it. *Merriam-Webster* defines apprehension as suspicion or fear, especially of future evil. Anxiety can be a protective biological response to danger, and it is ok to visit your doctor about your signs of anxiety. Your family physician may refer you to a psychiatrist who specializes in mental health issues like anxiety. If a person overreacts to their anxiety by thinking and doing things to harm themselves, then they should seek emergency medical care."

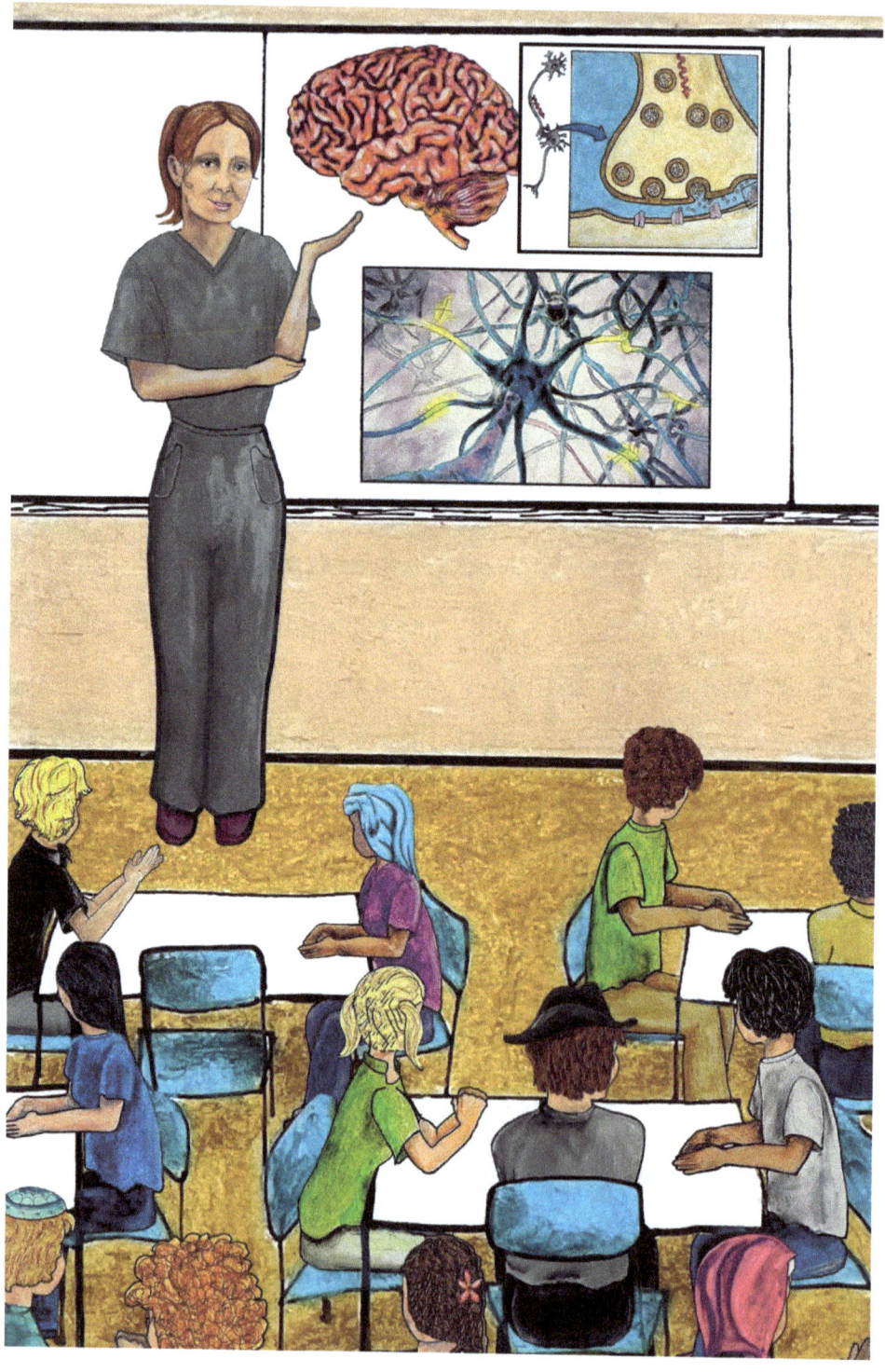

"The emotion of anxiety is based in the brain. Some people may feel unease in their stomach with high anxiety, but the feelings still originate in the brain. The brain has billions of neurons, and an example of a neuron is shown in the lower picture. A neuron can have thousands of connections with many other neurons, and they communicate with each other through the release of neurotransmitters to each other. A neurotransmitter then contacts the next neuron and causes an opening in the cell membrane so that certain chemicals rush inside via diffusion. An example of the end of a neuron is shown by the picture in the top right. The chemicals inside then add up to either cause the next neuron to send a signal or not send a signal. Sending a signal will then release neurotransmitters to the next neurons.

All feelings, including anxiety, are created by the mixture of neuronal signals to each other. Your environment helps create certain neuronal transmissions in your brain, and then your brain will react with certain emotions such as anxiety. The main neurotransmitters involved in anxiety are serotonin and norepinephrine. Feelings of anxiety can be seen on a spectrum where the experience may be very mild to extremely severe, resulting in a panic attack. Anxiety may include possible layers of fears of multiple threats in the environment that may be real or only perceived. The way to manage your anxiety is to combat it with a synergy of treatments. Synergism is defined by Merriam-Webster as interaction of discrete agencies, agents, or conditions such that the total effect is greater than the sum of the individual effects."

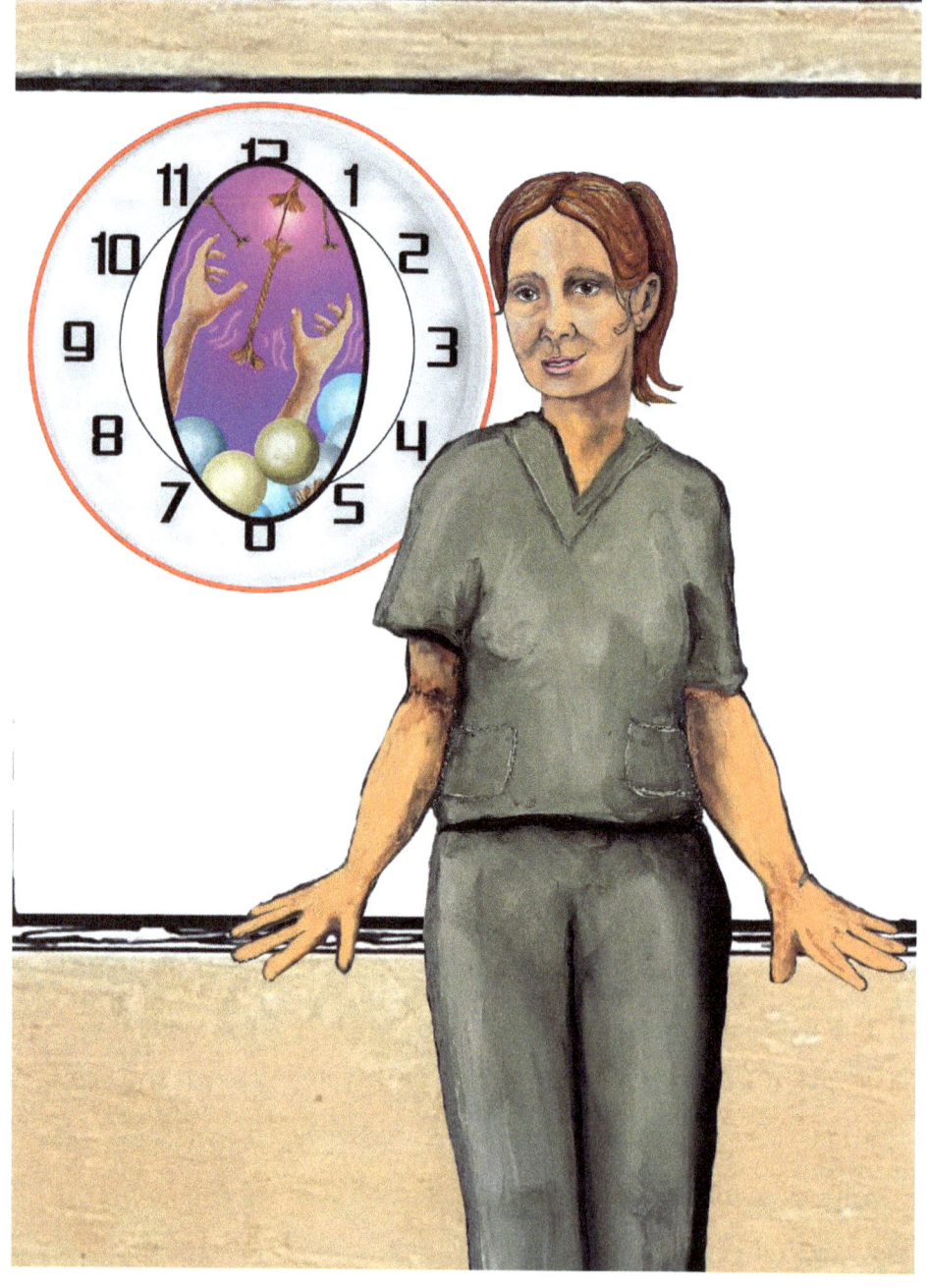

"Anxiety can be caused by a future event like being told that you will need to speak before a group of people. Anxiety can be caused by seeing a person. Seeing the person may be a trigger, since he or she may have done some very stressful things to you, so your brain expects the person to do more stressful things to you. Anxiety can also be caused by the environment, since a hurricane may cause a family to feel their home is in jeopardy of being destroyed. Anxiety is also caused by perception with no relation to reality, such as reading a horror fiction book and believing the characters in the story are about to be killed. Anxiety can be caused by a situation such as going to the doctor's office where you have previously received bad medical news from the doctor about your health.

Now, let's discuss with each other about a time when you were anxious. Share with those around you now, or write in your journal if you are doing the class by yourself. We'll let you share with the class as you feel comfortable afterwards."

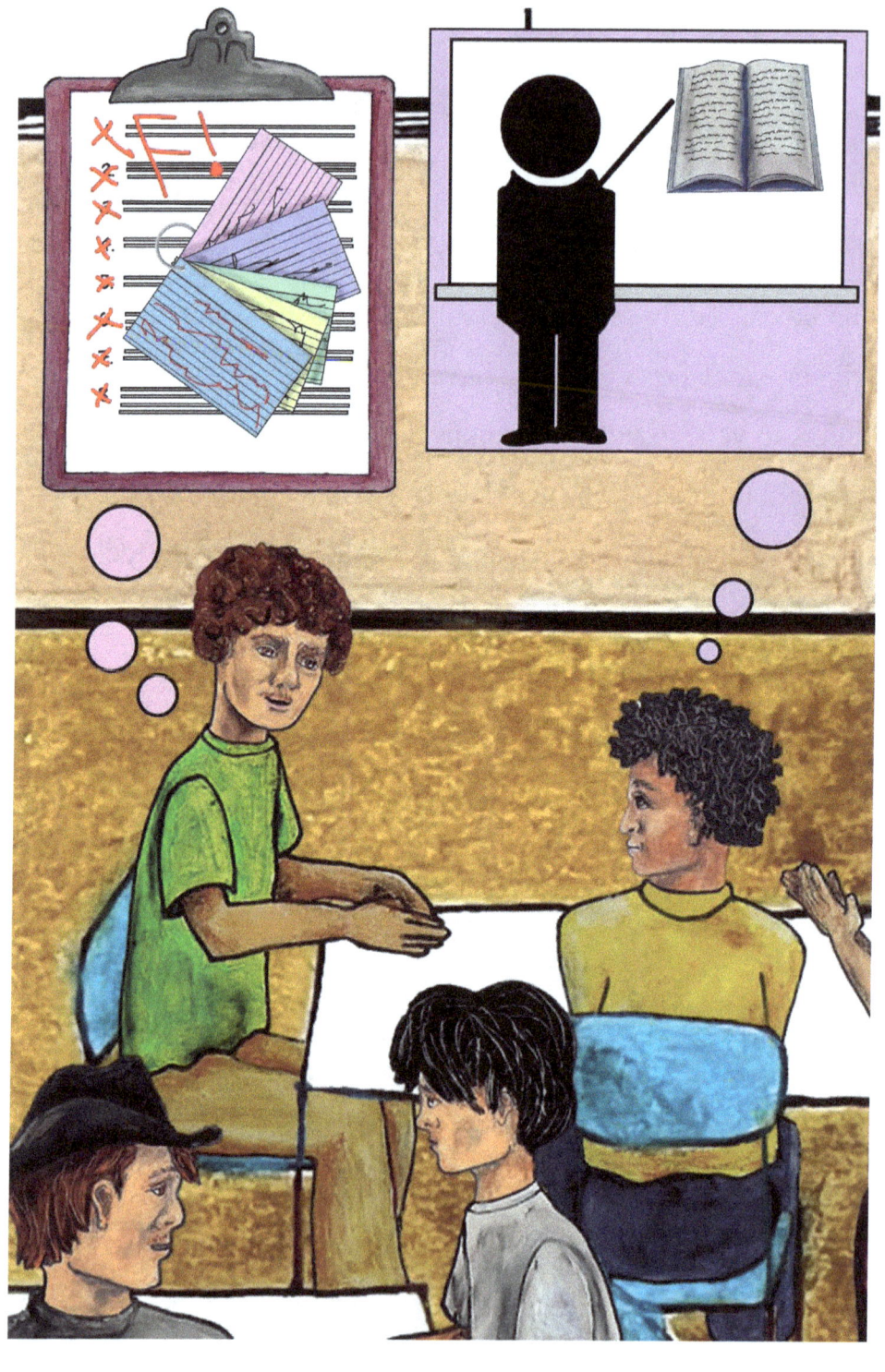

Gustavo raises his hand, and Nurse Dorothea calls on him to speak. "Once, I didn't study for a test and got it back from the teacher with a failing grade. The next time I went to the teacher's class for an exam, I was very anxious when I was given the exam papers, even though I had studied. The next day when the teacher was handing the exam papers back to the students, my heart was pounding, and I started to sweat a little. I got the papers back, and I passed. Now, when I get exam papers back from teachers, I still feel a little anxiety, but it isn't as strong as that other day, because I study for every test now."

"Thanks for sharing. One of the treatments for dealing with anxiety is preparing for the situation appropriately so that you can succeed at the task," says Nurse Dorothea.

Amari raises his hand, and Nurse Dorothea calls on him to speak. "Once, I was asked to talk in front of class about a book we were supposed to read. I had read it, but I felt my heart racing right before I was asked to stand in front of everyone. I told my teacher after class what I experienced, and they suggested making note cards about points I would want to share with a group and memorizing those cards. I did that the next time, and it really helped me gather my thoughts. I was still anxious before I spoke in front of everyone later in the course, but it seemed more manageable."

"Public speaking can be a great fear for many. Rehearsing your speech is a great way to manage your anxiety," says Nurse Dorothea.

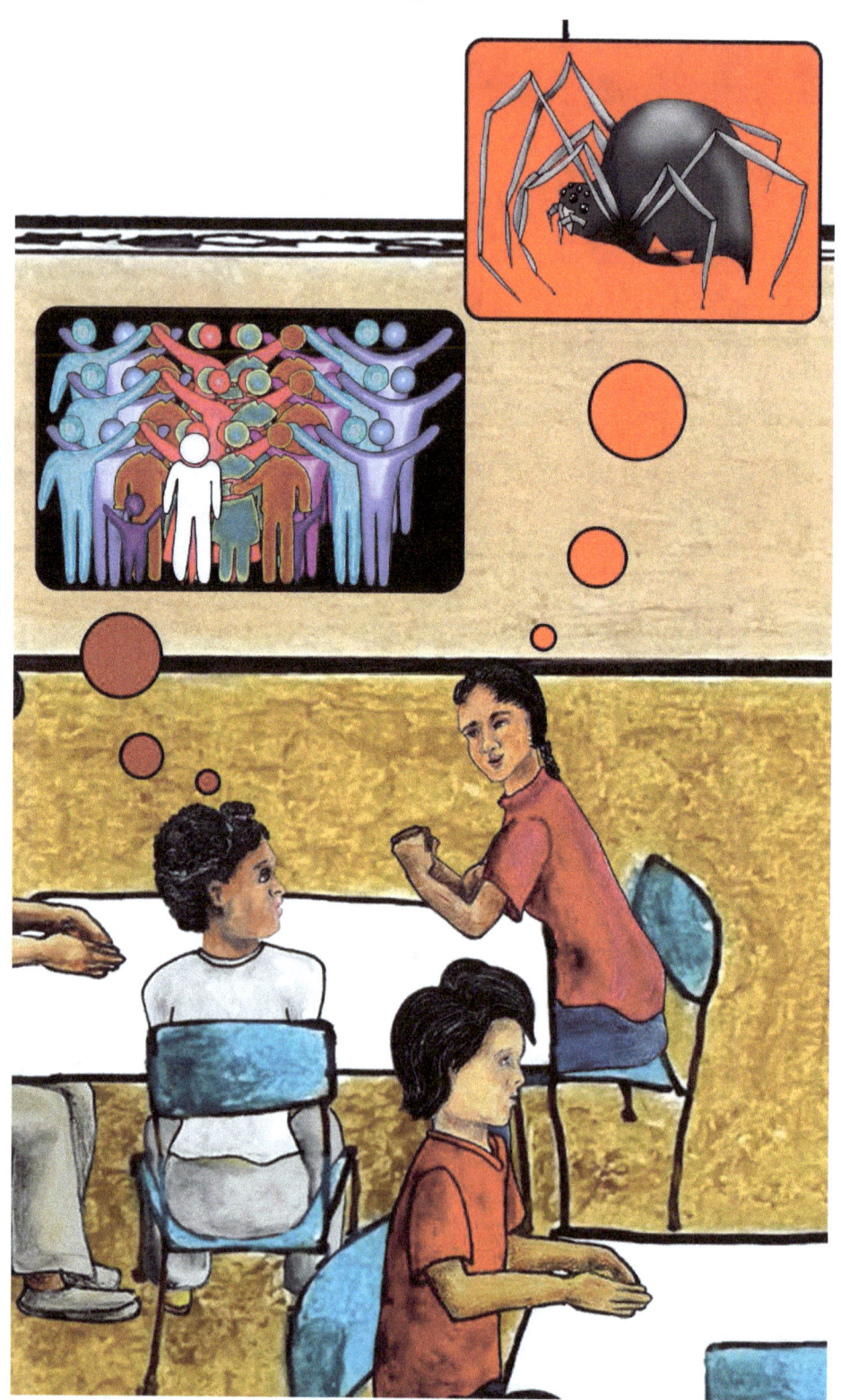

Amisha raises her hand, and Nurse Dorothea calls on her to speak. "Being in large groups makes me anxious because I don't think I'll stay safe. When my parents are with me, I feel less anxious since I believe they would protect me."

"It doesn't sound like your anxiety or fear of crowds is severe, but some people's anxiety can lead to extreme fear where the person stops doing activities of daily living. The irrational fear of crowds is called enochlophobia. Some people have to go through desensitization training, where they go into a small crowd and do coping skills in the middle of the crowd to help lower their anxiety. Later, they go into a larger crowd and continue practicing coping skills. Finally, after repeated training, they are able to go into a crowd and continue living their life," says Nurse Dorothea.

Pia raises her hand, and Nurse Dorothea calls on her to speak. "I'm afraid of spiders, and whenever I hear that one is in the room, I get really anxious. A couple of times, I have dreamed about them, and it turned into a nightmare where I woke up sweating."

"Some spiders can be very dangerous, like a black widow, so you want to avoid getting bitten by any spider. You are not alone in your concern about spiders. Spiders do have a use in the environment, and they help with lowering flying insect populations. Sometimes, seeing the use of something that we fear can help gain another perspective, so that we are not as fearful and are accepting of the living being's existence," says Nurse Dorothea.

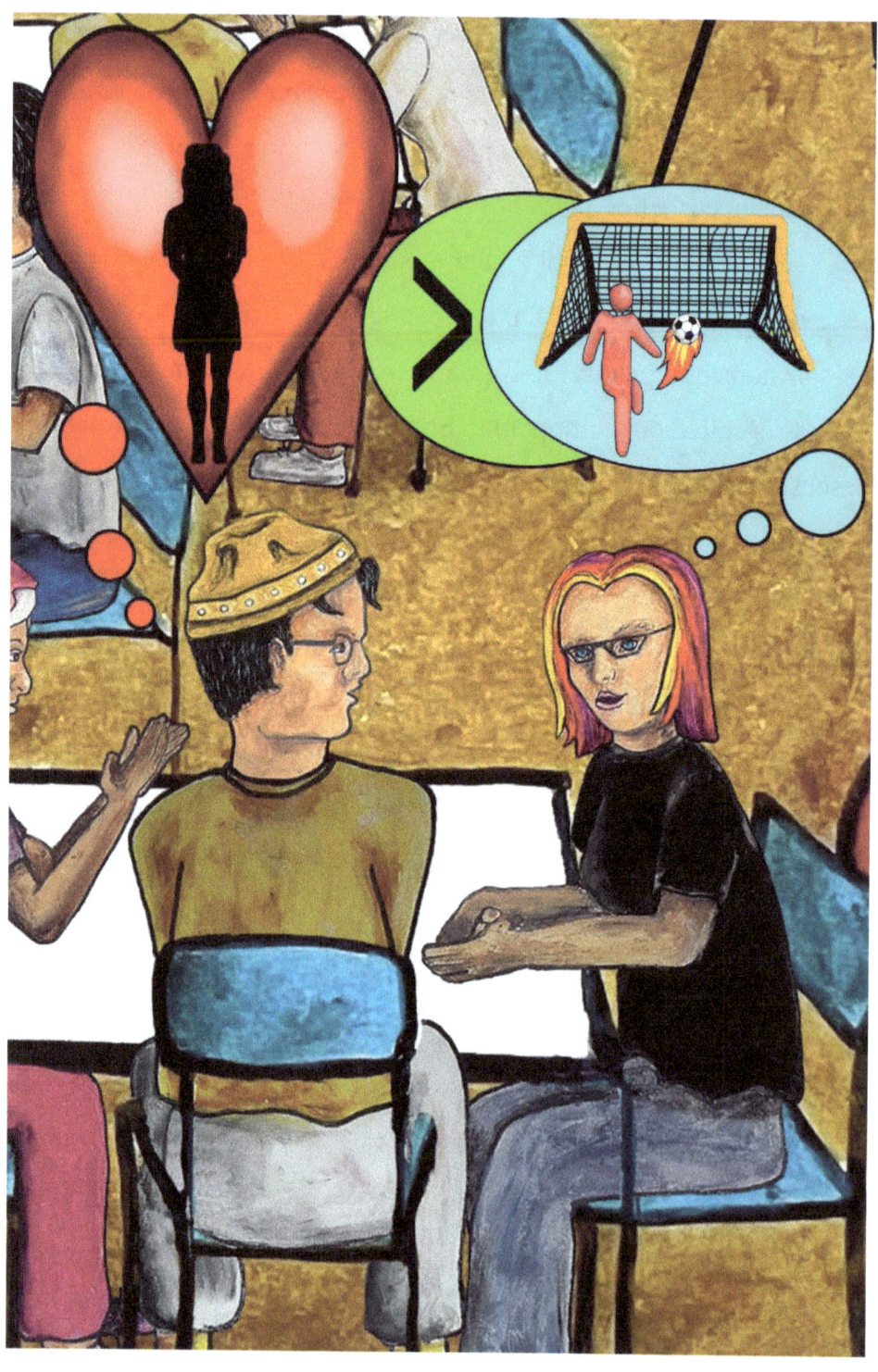

Azamat raises his hand, and Nurse Dorothea calls on him to speak. "There's a girl who I like, and when I think about walking up to her to start a conversation, I feel very anxious. It is keeping me from talking to her."

"Connecting with another person in a romantic way can be scary because of the uncertainty of how the relationship will turn out. It is part of human existence to start friendships with strangers since we were all strangers, at one point to our friends. A romantic relationship takes courage, and doing things despite your anxiety is sometimes needed to start something that could last a lifetime," says Nurse Dorothea.

Juniper raises her hand, and Nurse Dorothea calls on her to speak. "I love to play soccer, and I'm really good at it, but when we went to the state championship tournament last year, I was very anxious before the game started. I didn't want to let my teammates down and make a mistake. Once we started playing, I got more comfortable and just focused on doing my best at every moment. I even helped score a goal."

"Whenever we have a high-stakes event, it can create anxiety since we realize we only have one chance to do it correctly. Living moment by moment and doing the best you can is a great way to deal with your anxiety in high-stakes environments. When you know you did your best, you can sleep more easily that night, whatever the outcome, although a disappointing outcome can create other challenging emotions," says Nurse Dorothea.

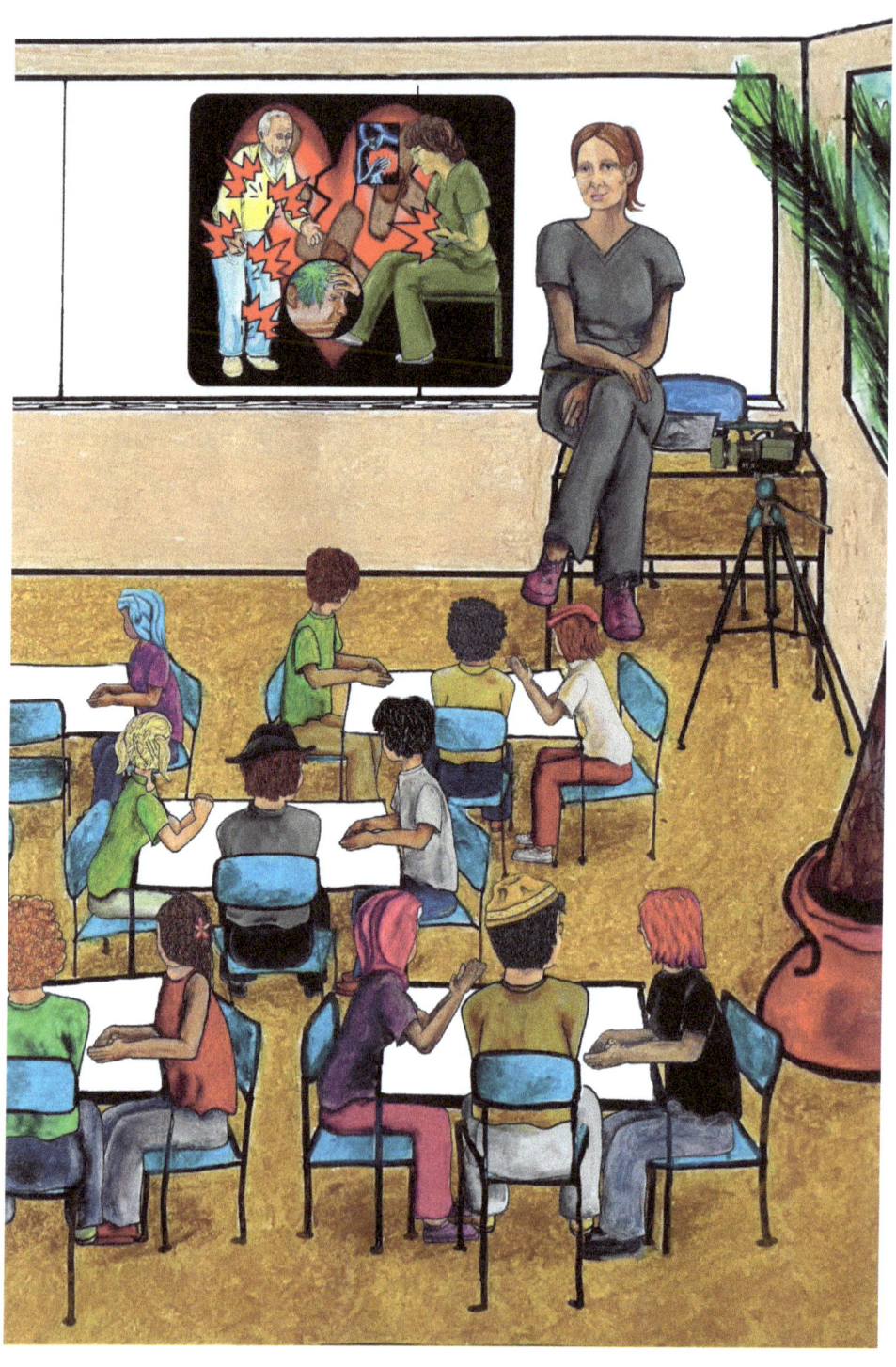

"People can get physical symptoms from this mental health challenge. Physical manifestations of anxiety can be headache, stomachache, muscle tension, tiredness, rapid heartbeat, shortness of breath, dizziness, sweaty palms, trembling hands or legs, fast breathing, upset stomach, clenched jaw, dry mouth, nausea, diarrhea, lightheadedness, and chest tightening. Some people get more than one symptom for an anxiety-producing event, and some may only get one. Some people's symptoms may be severe enough for them to seek emergency medical care, and others may take an over-the-counter medication to help, such as a calcium tablet for upset stomach. The number of symptoms can be on a spectrum and the severity of the symptoms can be on a spectrum."

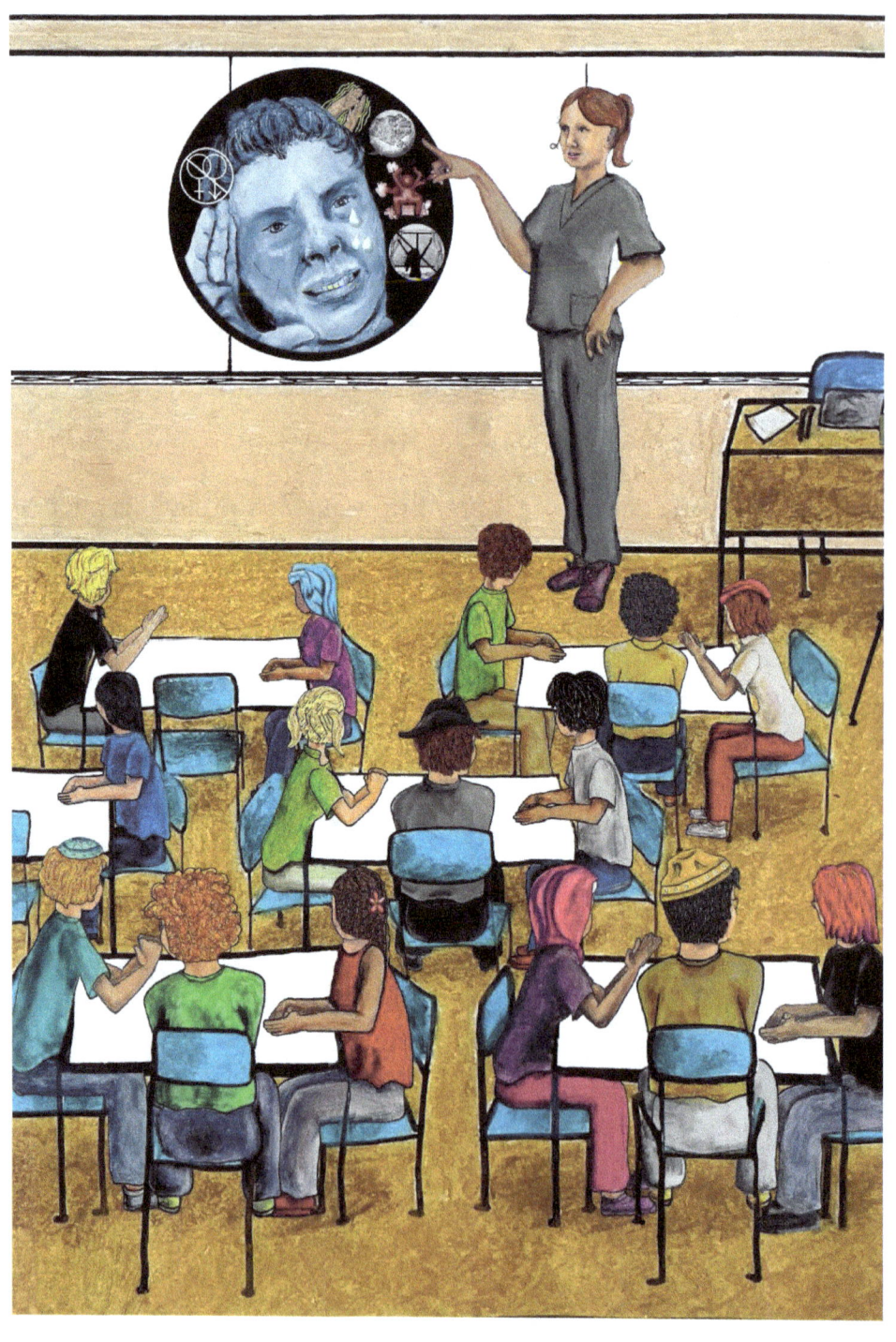

"There can also be mental symptoms of anxiety such as trouble concentrating, self-consciousness, nervousness, restlessness, distraction, feeling of having a heart attack or stroke, feelings of apprehension and fear, sleep problems, exaggerated feelings of dread, memory problems, fatigue, irritation, agitation, trouble making decisions, and sexual dysfunction. Just like physical symptoms, people's mental symptoms of anxiety can be on a spectrum, along with the number of mental symptoms, as well as the severity of the symptoms. Each anxiety-producing event can be unique in its number of symptoms and severity of symptoms."

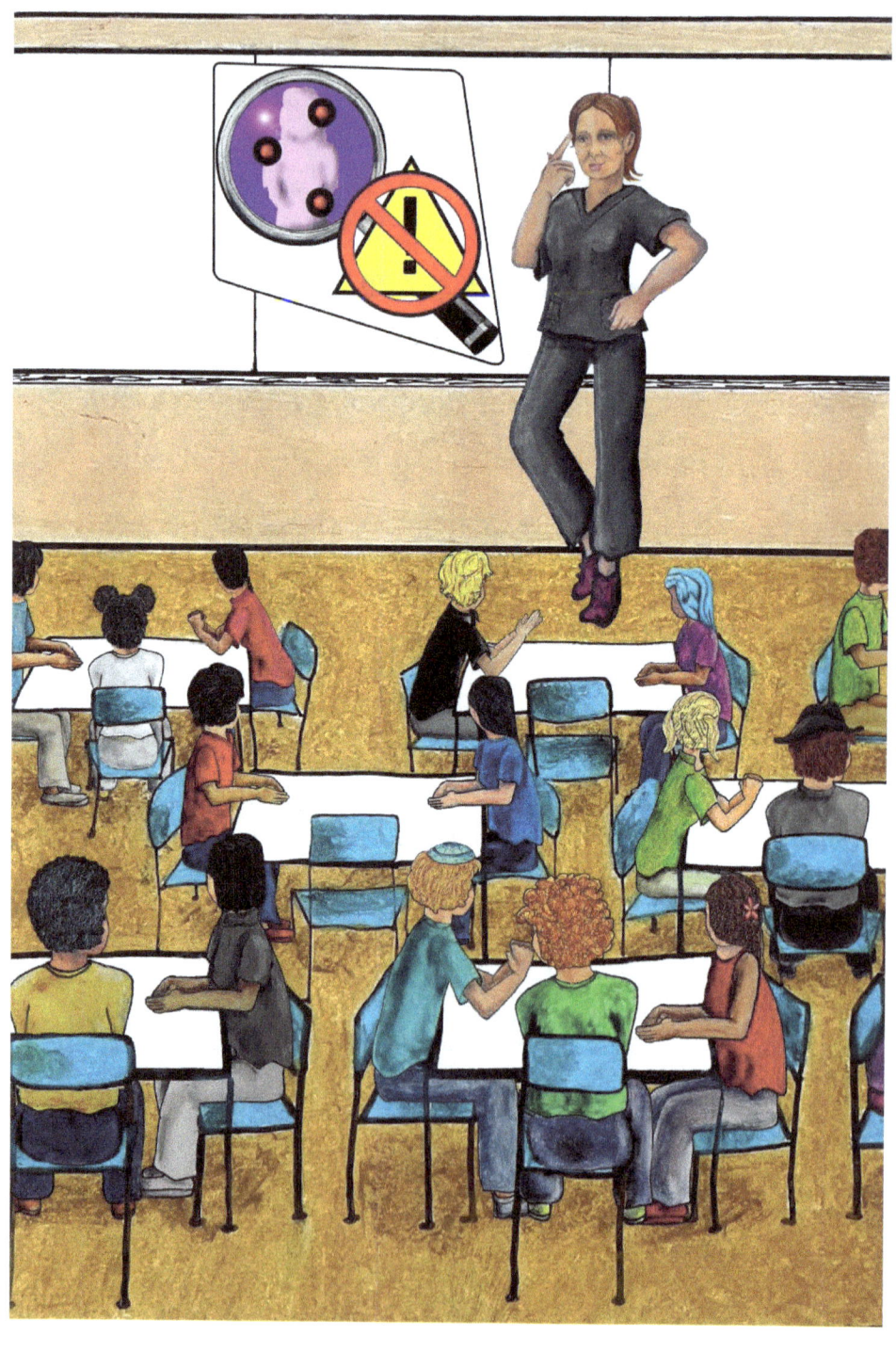

"Anxiety symptoms are not dangerous except for situations such as having trouble concentrating if you are driving a car and crash. People can learn to tolerate their symptoms. Try using the perspective that both physical and mental symptoms are a sign to take action. Each action may be different for each anxiety-producing event. The action may involve taking medication for your physical symptom. The action could involve engaging in a coping skill such as deep breathing. Try to allow yourself to tolerate the symptoms at a level where the symptoms are not too intense nor too suppressed. Learning to live with a level of distress is a skill called distress tolerance.

You shouldn't avoid all scenarios that produce anxiety. Try not to limit your life activities just so that you won't experience anxiety. It's important, so I'll say it again. Try not to limit your life activities just so that you won't experience anxiety, because it is an emotion that can be managed using layers of healthy coping skills. Some people need to do many different coping skills over a period of time, and some need to do many coping skills at the same time to produce a unique effect. If your coping skill is not successful, it doesn't mean it didn't work at all, but you may need to do other things or do something for a longer period of time, such as deep breathing for five minutes instead of one minute."

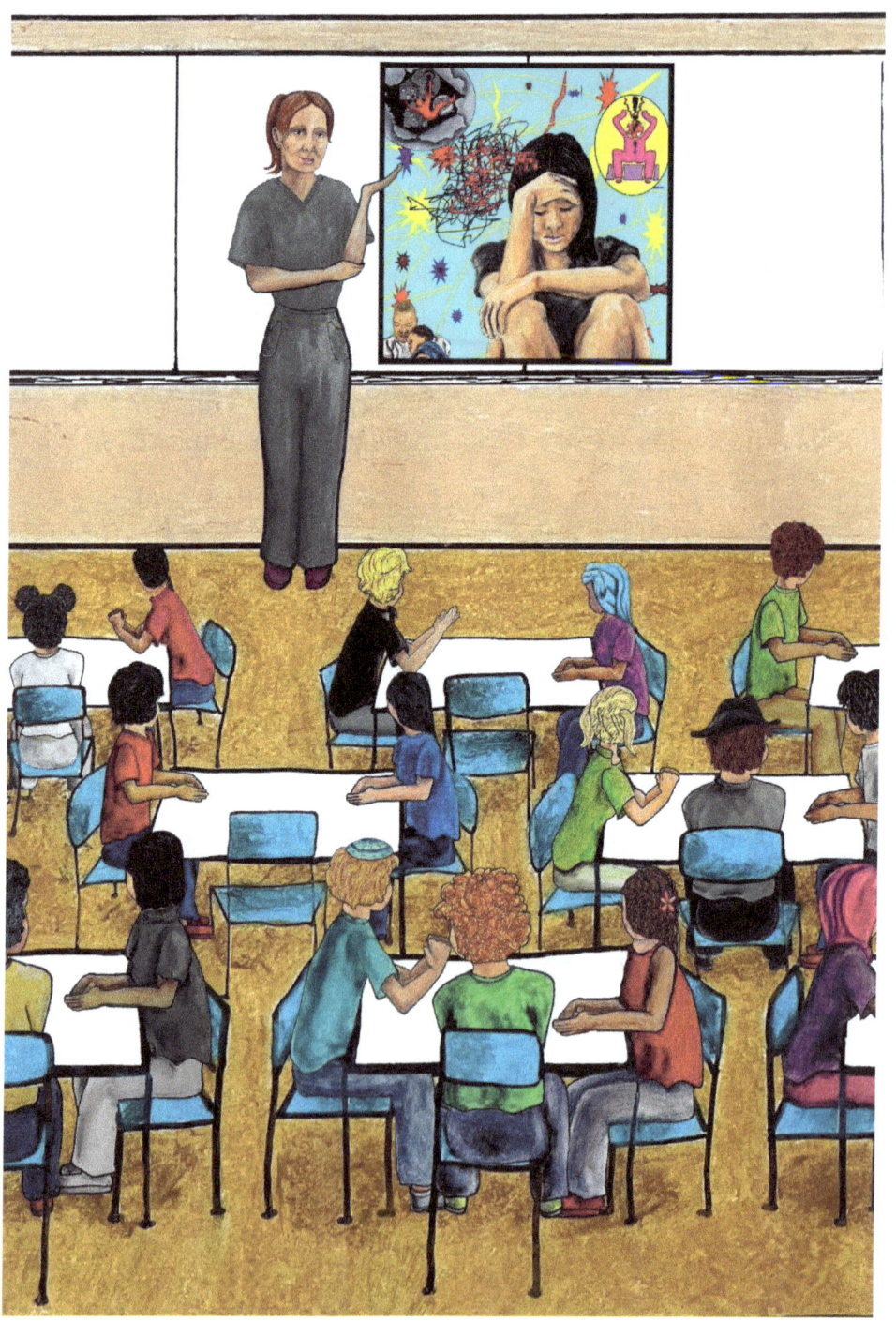

"Some people's anxiety needs to be treated by a psychiatrist. Some examples are generalized anxiety disorder, post-traumatic stress disorder or PTSD, and postpartum anxiety. It is ok to ask for help. Some women may experience a lot of anxiety during pregnancy due to all of the unknowns that may be coming, such as what the baby will look like, will they be able to provide adequately for the baby's future, will the baby be healthy, and will they be able to get the resources they need to help the baby mature into a strong and happy adult. Some people may experience acute stress disorder, where something or many things may happen that cause severe anxiety. With support from the treatment team, people can regain their mental equilibrium and return to a baseline level of functioning that is acceptable."

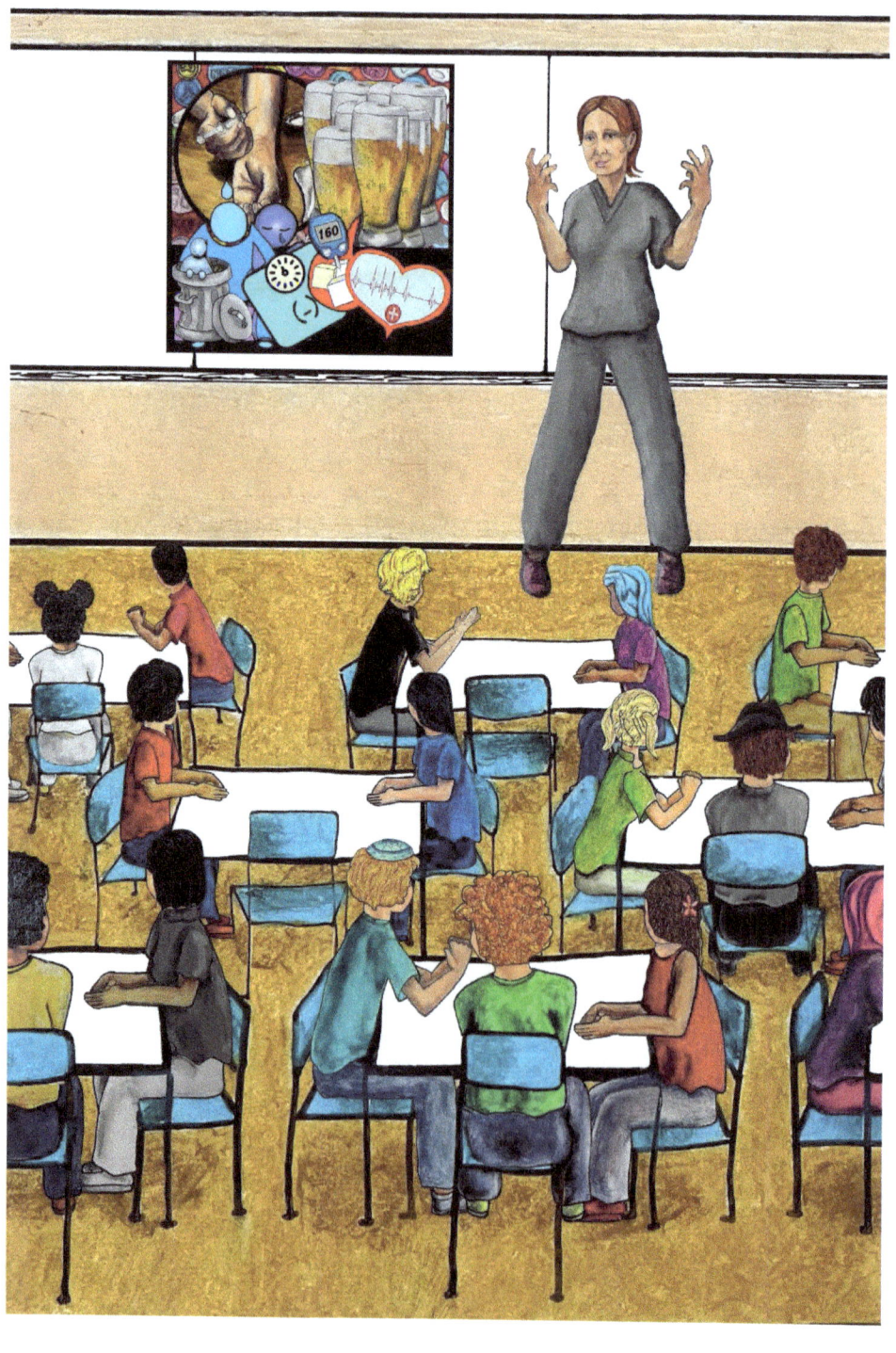

"Anxiety can cause complications. Some people's anxiety can lead them to develop depression since they may think they may not be able to overcome the anxiety and live well with their circumstances. Some people turn to substance abuse to get a temporary fix. Substance abuse can lead to addiction, and the path of recovery can be difficult for some people. Some people develop low self-esteem, since they think they are managing their life improperly.

Anxiety can also lead to insecurity, which can impact relationships. Some medical complications of anxiety can be heart disease, stroke, type 2 diabetes, and low birth weight for children born to mothers dealing with high anxiety. You are a valued member of society, and we need you to operate at your best, so that you can give the most back to your culture. Getting the help you need early in anxiety management can lead to successful outcomes. Also, encourage your family and friends to get the help they may need if you see something wrong."

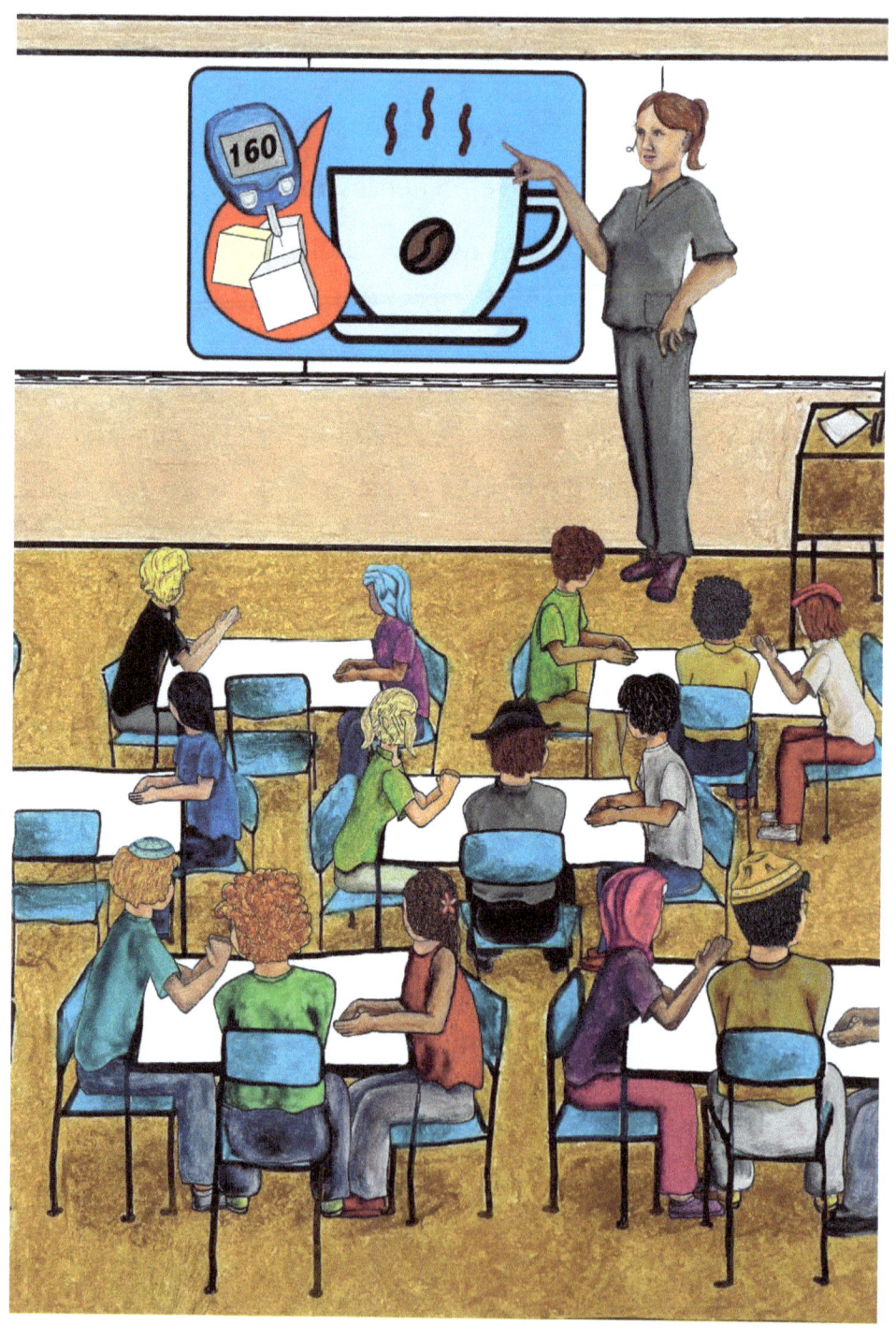

"Some things that can exacerbate symptoms are sugar and caffeine. If you notice that you are dealing with regular high levels of anxiety, observe if your consumption of either or both sugar and caffeine is high. If one or both is high in your diet, consider reducing the amount, and see if that helps you get to a tolerable level of anxiety. Let's switch gears and discuss a technique that helps with a lot of mental health challenges. Listing triggers can be very helpful since this activity helps create insight into your mind.

Now, let's all write down on a piece of paper all your triggers that you have noticed, which are anxiety-producing events. After you have spent some time writing the list, share some of your insights with those around you, and then we'll let you share with the class as you feel comfortable. Let's do this activity now. If you are reading this book or watching the video, write a list like the others in the classroom are doing, too."

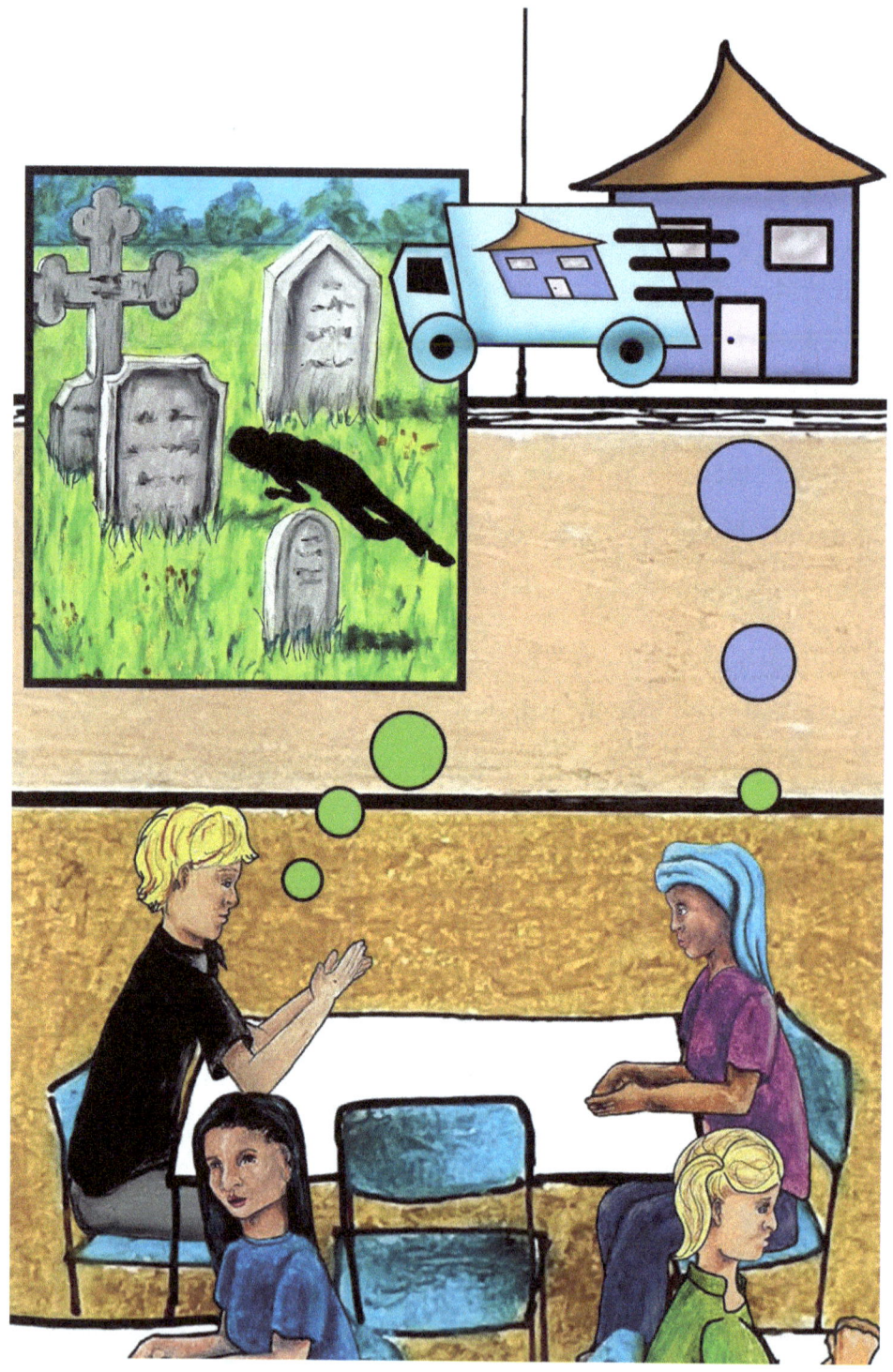

Dimitry raises his hand, and Nurse Dorothea calls on him to speak. "One of my triggers is the death of a loved one. Anytime it happens, I get anxious and start thinking about my own mortality."

"Facing our own death can cause anxiety for all humans. No one on Earth has escaped anxiety from thinking about their death. Let us choose a path of responding to our mortality with courage instead of fear, and create a plan of action to better ourselves as well as the world with the little time we have left in it," says Nurse Dorothea.

Yulianna raises her hand, and Nurse Dorothea calls on her to speak. "Something on my list is moving to a new apartment. My family has not had physical home security, and every time we have to move into a different home, I get anxious."

"Physical security, such as having a place to call home is part of Maslow's hierarchy of needs. If our basic needs are not met, then we can experience a mental health challenge such as anxiety. Some social workers can help families with home security, so it's always a good idea to ask for social assistance if it is needed, such as getting referrals for financial management classes or assistance with making monthly payments. Learning to live within our earned income is important, and it would be better to live in a smaller home that could be permanent instead of trying to live in a larger place. Changing homes is a big deal for children since it may also involve changing schools, which can be very disruptive," says Nurse Dorothea.

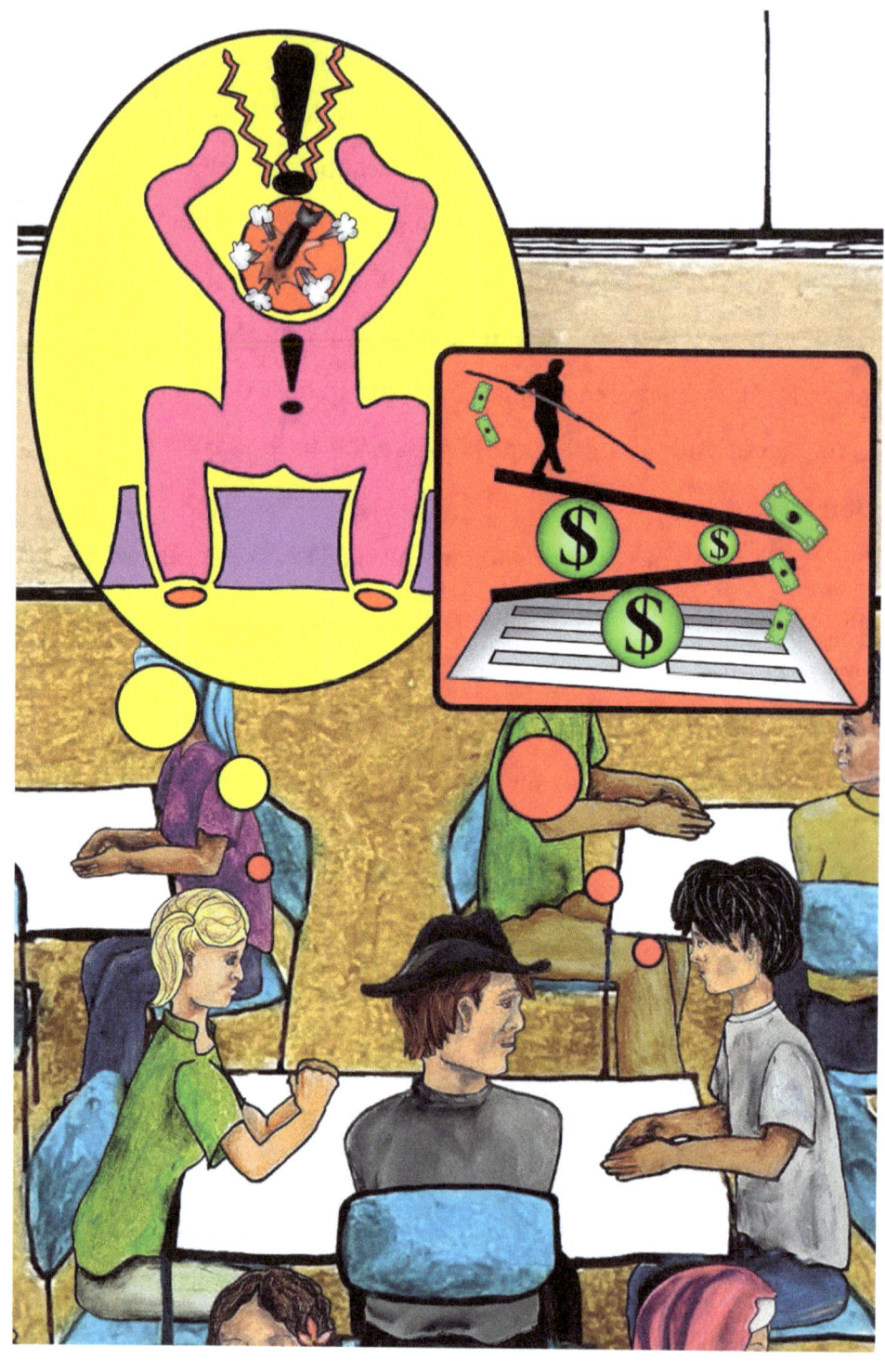

Frida raises her hand, and Nurse Dorothea calls on her to speak. "Something on my list is a reminder of my PTSD event. Every time I'm in a certain place, my symptoms happen. Just thinking about going to certain places can cause me to be anxious, because I know my PTSD symptoms will happen once I get there."

"PTSD can be debilitating for some, and people experiencing PTSD may need psychiatric services. If your mental health challenge is causing you difficulty in completing your activities of daily living, then you should seek professional mental health services," says Nurse Dorothea.

Antonio raises his hand, and Nurse Dorothea calls on him to speak. "When I hear my parents talking about their money problems, it causes me anxiety since I know that when they start talking about it in front of us, it means things are going to get bad, and we won't be able to do all the things we want to do. It may also mean a lot of eating cheap foods for a couple of months."

"Some communities have special projects, such as a community garden, so that people in need can get food. Some communities have non-profit organizations which provide free boxes of food each month, and others may have special food markets, so that people can buy excess fruits and vegetables at a deep discount, so that the food doesn't spoil. Families should reach out to social workers in the community, so that they can get info about what is available for their food insecurity," says Nurse Dorothea.

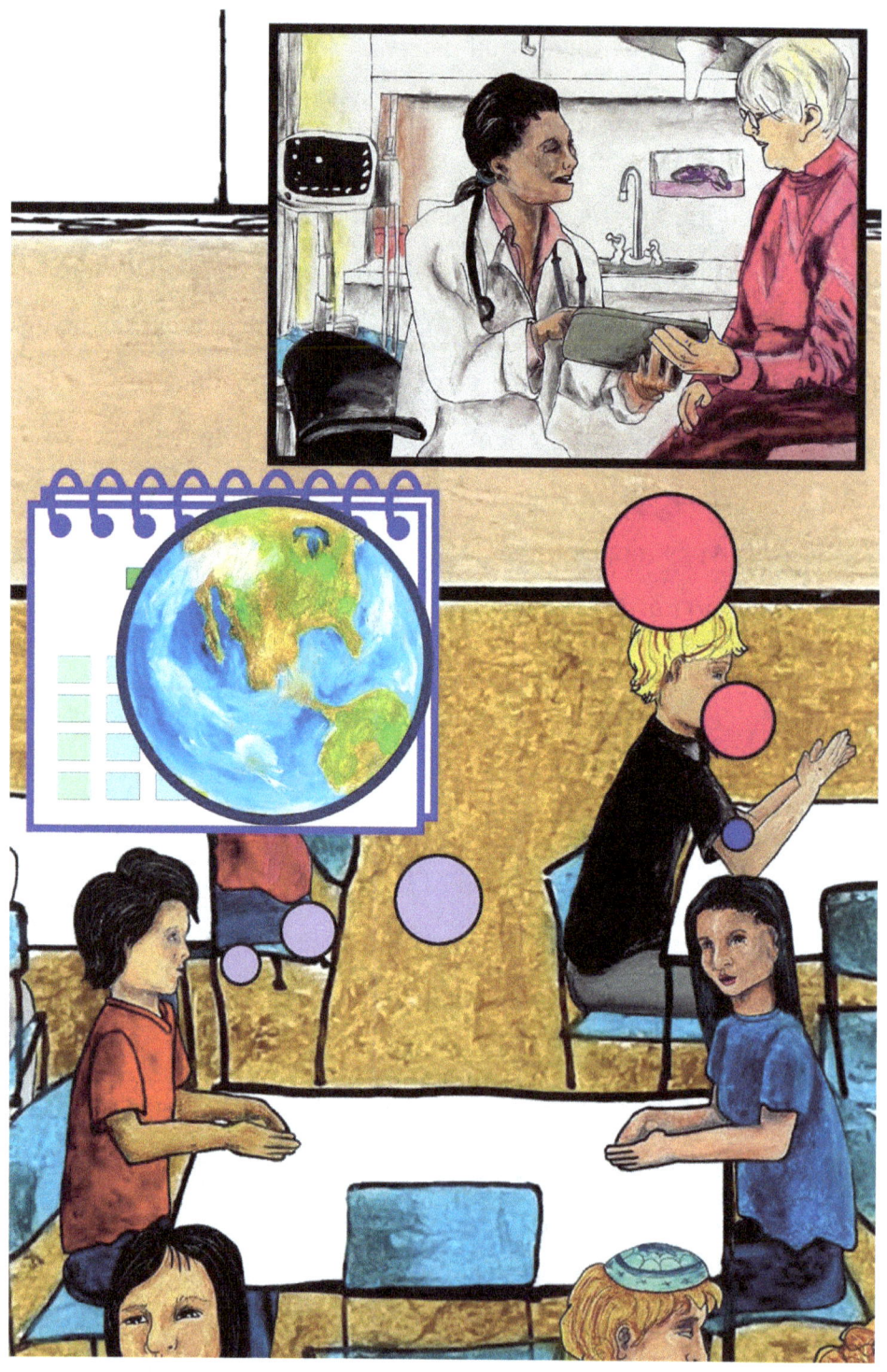

Kenji raises his hand, and Nurse Dorothea calls on him to speak. "I'm from a country that went through a civil war, and a lot of innocent people were killed. Whenever I hear about world events discussing war, it makes me anxious since I am familiar with some events that kids will experience in those areas."

"War is awful, and we should do everything in our power to prevent it," says Nurse Dorothea.

Diwa raises her hand, and Nurse Dorothea calls on her to speak. "When I get health check-ups, I get really anxious the day before and the morning of the appointment. I haven't shared this with many people, but I was diagnosed with a childhood cancer when I was 8 years old. I had a team of great doctors and nurses who brought me through it, but I still get very anxious every time I see my doctor and fear that she may tell me that the cancer has come back."

"When people get diseases, it can affect them for the rest of their lives. I'm sorry to hear that you went through that. Thanks for being brave enough to share your struggle with us. I trust you have a strong support network that helps you," says Nurse Dorothea.

"I do. My mom always takes a vacation day from work to go to my appointments with me, and my uncle sends me nice text messages the day before and the day of my visit. I also have a great support group of other kids who have battled cancer, and they encourage me as well," says Diwa.

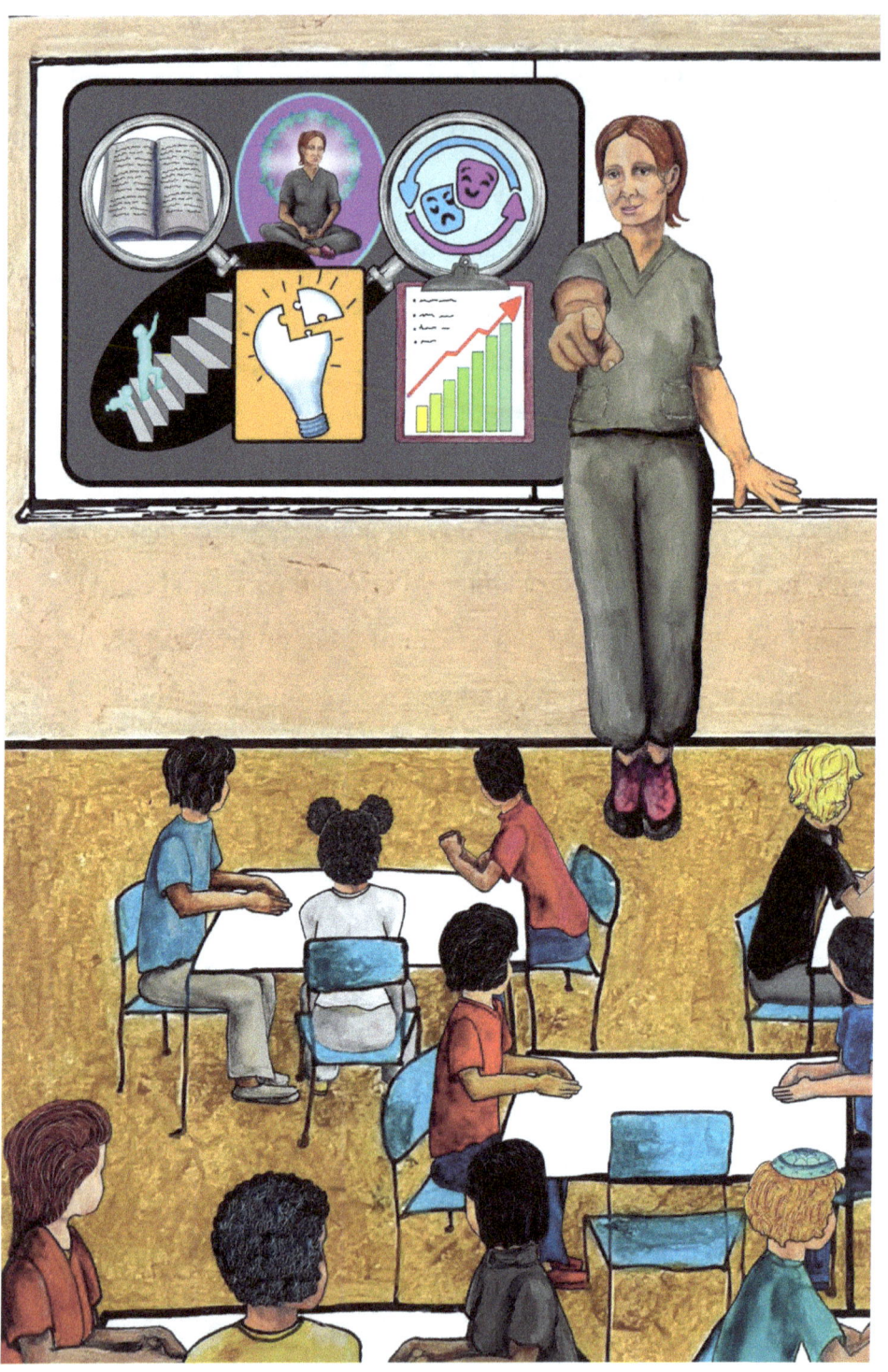

"Self-regulation is necessary to manage anxiety. *Merriam-Webster* defines self-regulation as control or supervision from within instead of by an external authority. Many different types of knowledge and skills are needed for successful self-regulation. A person should educate themselves on emotions, and learn to identify each of their emotions when they are having them. A person should learn to self-soothe, instead of depending on someone else to soothe them or bring them back to peace. A person should learn perspective-taking, which can also be called the ability to walk in another person's shoes. When you can learn to see things from someone else's perspective, it helps you apply different perspectives to your situation.

A person should learn many different social skills such as taking turns to use a resource, practicing patience with another person so that you can give yourself patience, paying attention to another person when they are talking so you can remain focused on something when it is needed, and problem solving with others so that you can learn to problem solve on your own. A person should learn to think flexibly, develop time management skills, and learn to set goals. Doing these things can help you face anxiety head on."

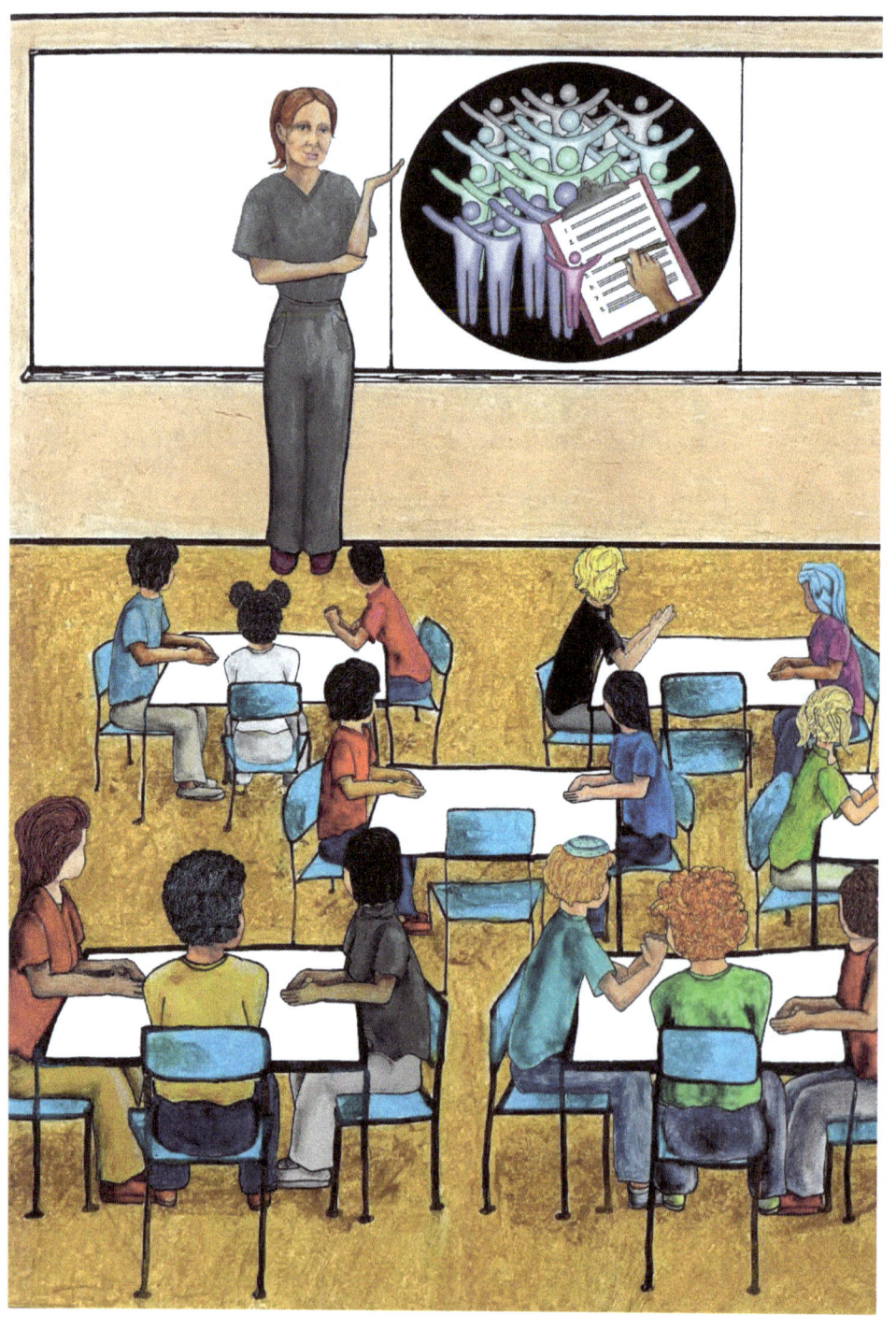

"Cognitive behavioral therapy, or CBT, is the gold standard for treatment of people with anxiety disorders. The main principle of CBT is that psychological problems are partly due to unhelpful ways of thinking, with learned patterns of unhelpful behaviors. People can learn more helpful ways of thinking and new behaviors so that they can be more effective in their life. CBT treatment involves recognizing distorted thinking, gaining insight into your behaviors and motivation of other people, learning to problem solve so you can handle difficult situations, and developing more confidence into one's own abilities. The CBT strategy involves facing one's fears, role-playing, and rehearsing difficult interactions so that you are better prepared for them, learning to calm one's mind, and relaxing one's body. In the USA, a CBT therapist can be found online at www.abct.org or www.adaa.org."

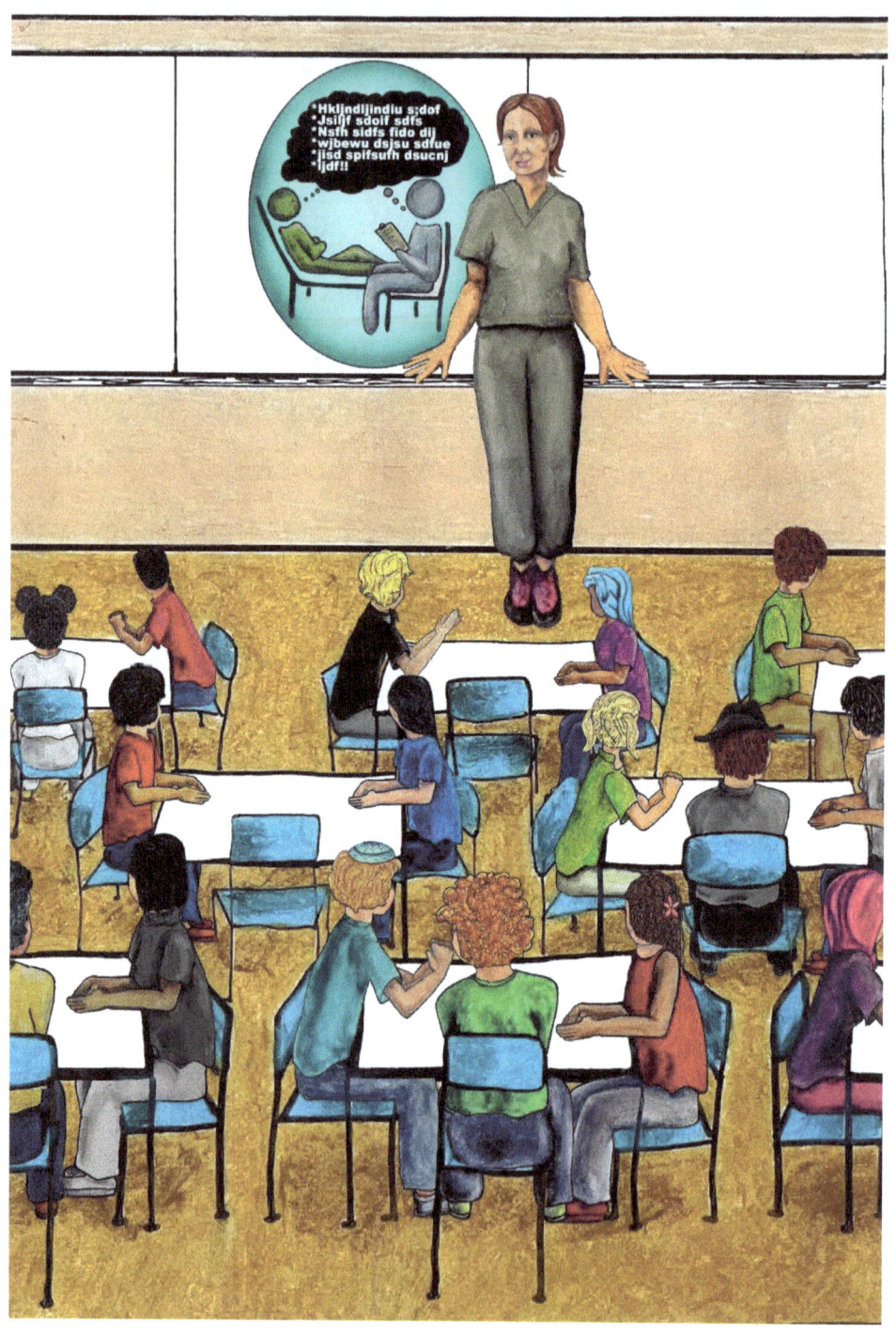

"Another type of psychological treatment that is helpful for anxiety is called psychodynamic therapy. A therapist will try to help the person discover the history behind the symptoms, and help examine the interpersonal conflicts that the person may be having with others, so they can address what is causing the anxiety."

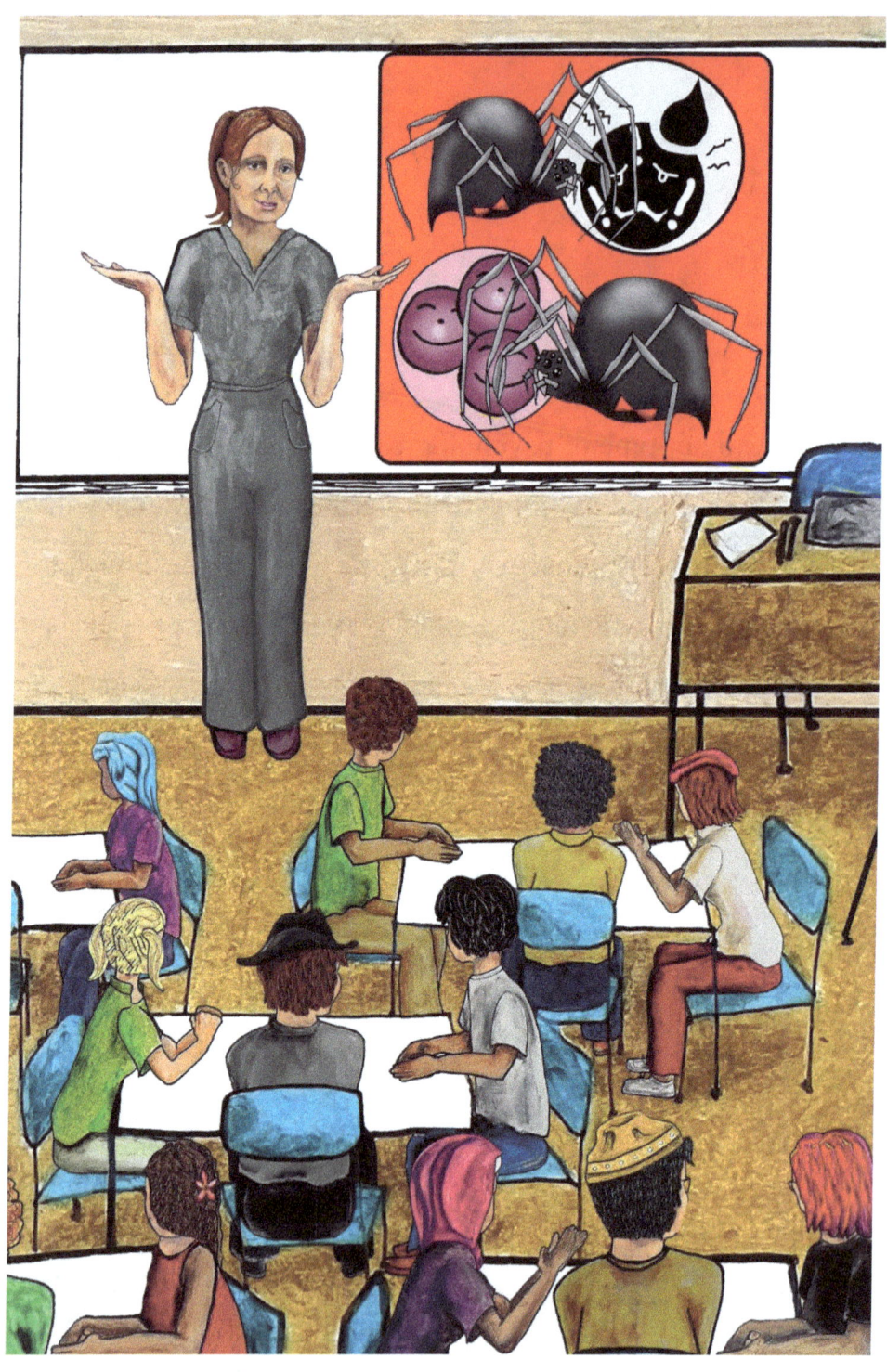

"Anxiety can also be treated with exposure and desensitization therapy. This is where the person is exposed to the anxiety-producing event. They may be exposed to a lesser form of the event and then led up to full exposure of the complete event that causes the anxiety. Distress tolerance is taught during the therapy, and coping skills are used during the events, so that the event no longer produces the extreme anxiety that it once did. People can find support groups regarding some of their anxiety-producing situations, so that they find the encouragement that they need and deserve. When anxiety prevents a person from doing activities of daily living, they need extra support, usually from people, so they can live a productive and happy life."

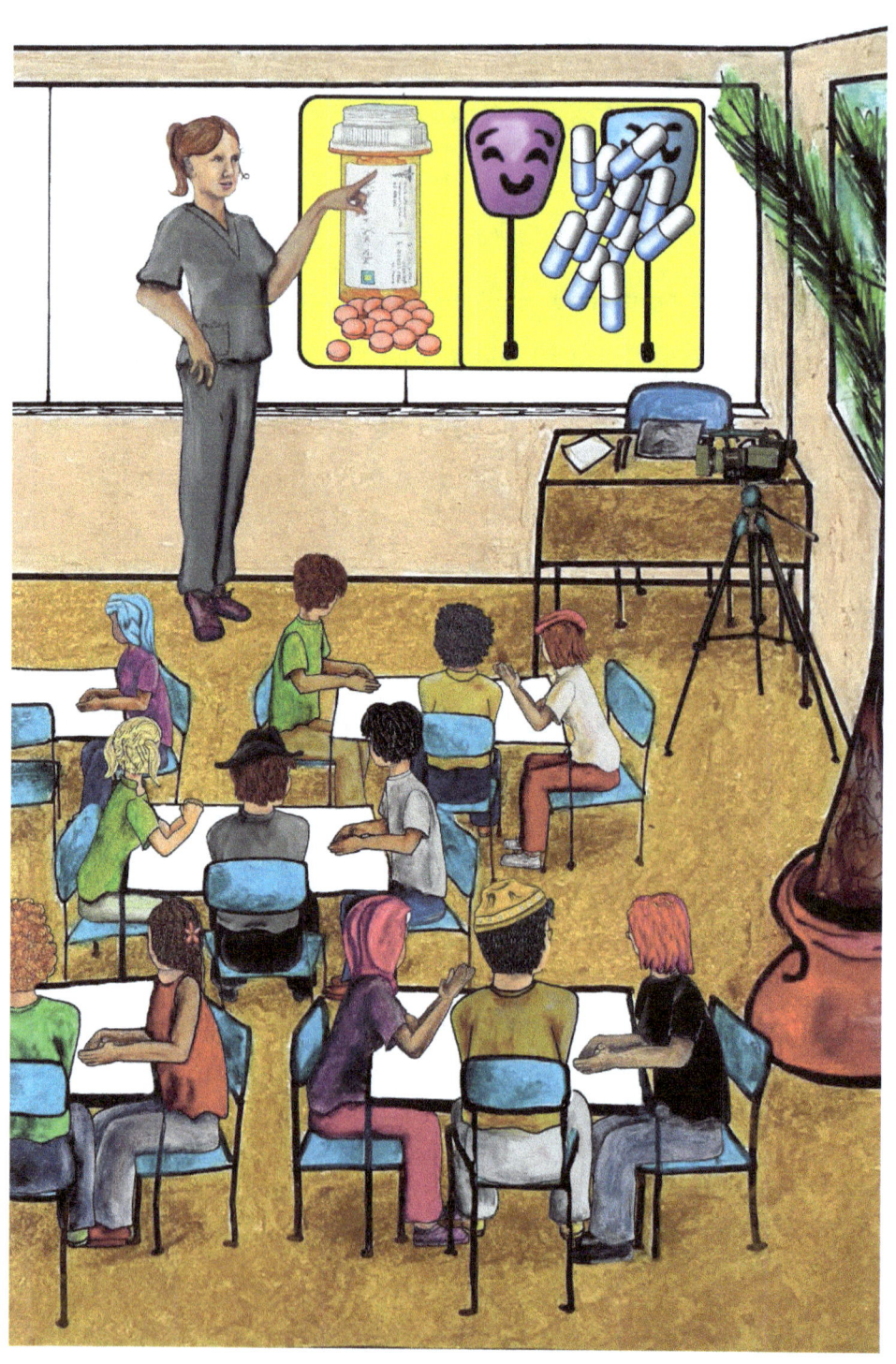

"When some people meet with a psychiatrist, they may be prescribed medication to help. Some people are given something called a beta blocker which can be propranolol. This medication has the ability to affect pulse and blood pressure though, so take only as prescribed. A person might be prescribed a benzodiazepine, which can be taken as needed for severe anxiety in certain situations. This medication can become addictive, and there can be seizures if a person takes it daily and stops abruptly, so take only as prescribed. Anti-depressants can be used for the long-term treatment of anxiety. Anti-depressants may need to be taken for 4-6 weeks before the full effect is achieved, so also take these only as prescribed."

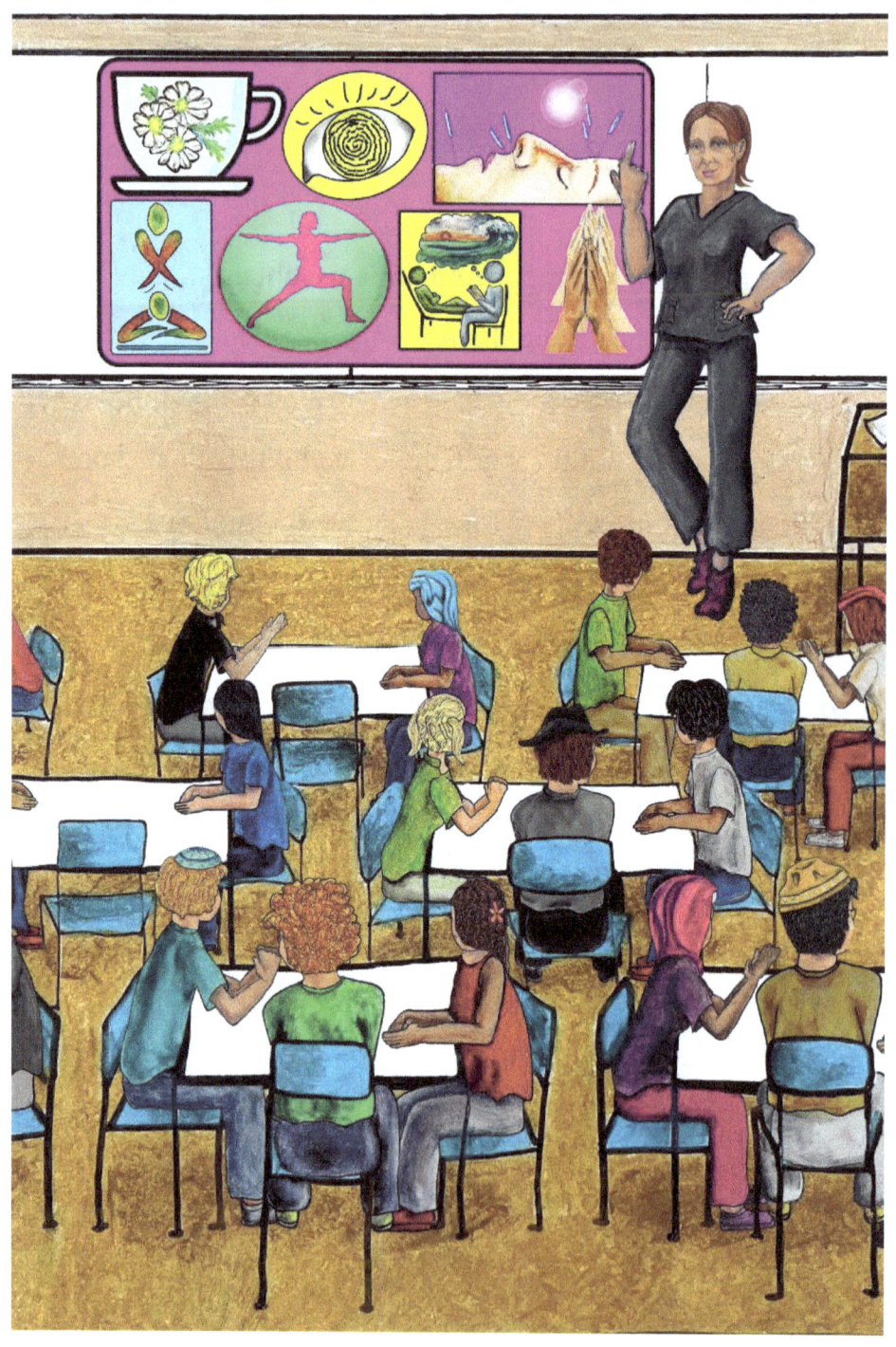

"Another therapy that could be tried is drinking chamomile tea. Some research shows this tea is effective in relaxing people. Some alternative therapies that some people find effective are hypnosis and acupuncture. There still needs to be more research conducted to confirm the usefulness of these approaches. Some people feel less anxious and relaxed after getting a massage, doing yoga, or putting a weighted blanket on their shoulders. Guided imagery is a therapy where a person is asked to close their eyes, and another person uses words to guide them to a different location in their mind, such as the beach or the forest. This type of therapy has been found to be helpful with increasing feelings of peace. Some religious people report feeling less anxious by doing repetitive prayers. Other people say mantras or repeat a word or simple sentence, and they report feeling less anxious after their meditation. Smelling lavender oil may also help you."

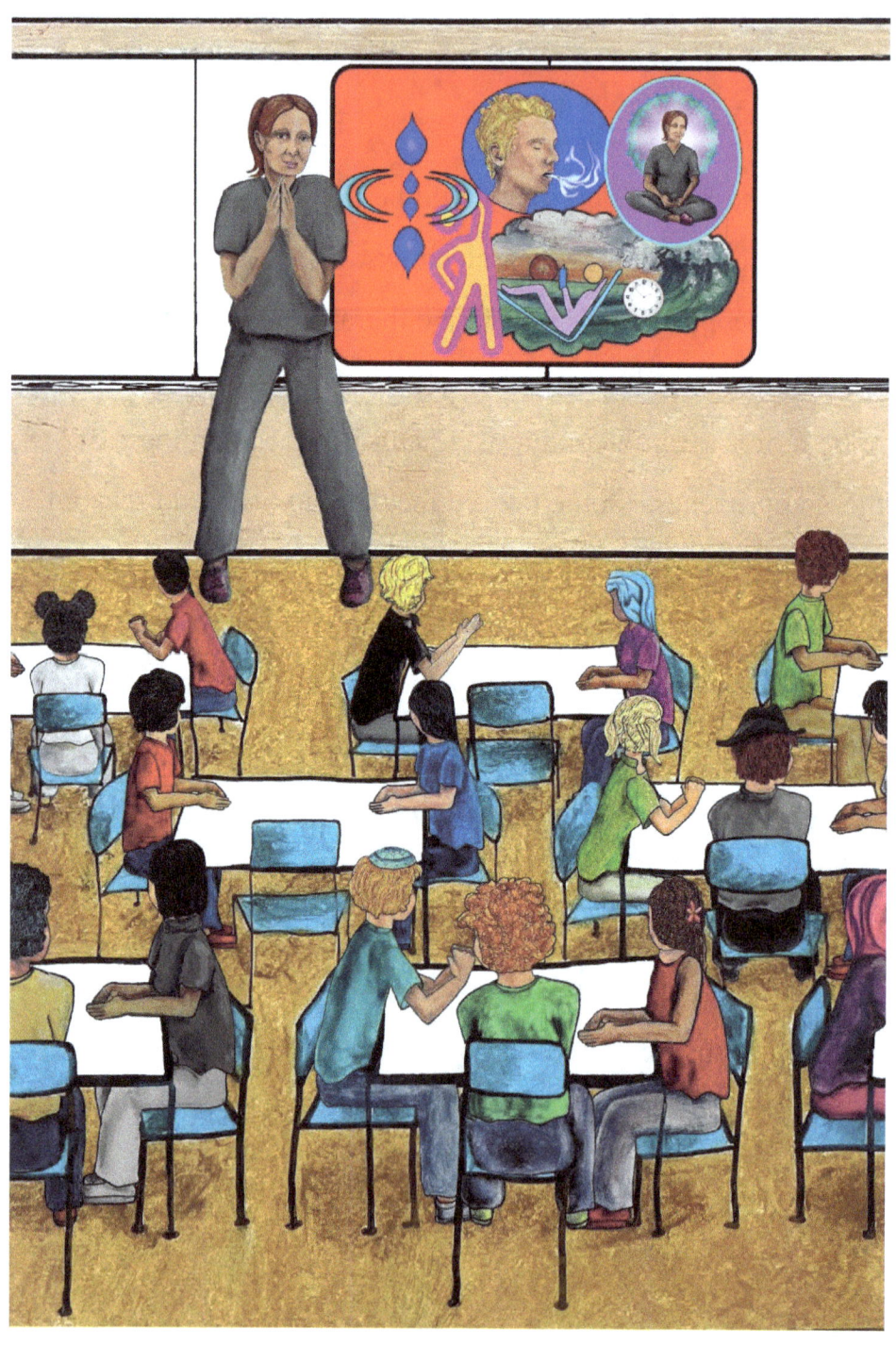

"Deep breathing has been found to be very effective for many people to reduce their anxiety levels to a tolerable level. Square breathing can be used where the person breathes in through their nose slowly for four seconds, holds their breath for four seconds, breathes out of their mouth for four seconds, and then doesn't breathe for four seconds. The cycle is repeated for at least two minutes. Some research shows that if a person meditates for 45 minutes a day, that can help reduce anxiety. It can also be helpful to meditate for 2.5 hours once a week with an instructor.

Mindfulness has been found to reduce anxiety, and it involves being aware of the present moment. *Merriam-Webster* defines mindfulness as the practice of maintaining a nonjudgmental state or heightened or complete awareness of one's thoughts, emotions, or experience on a moment-to-moment basis. Stretching exercises can help a person reduce their anxiety. Doing progressive muscle relaxation, where each muscle is contracted and then relaxed, can help lower anxiety."

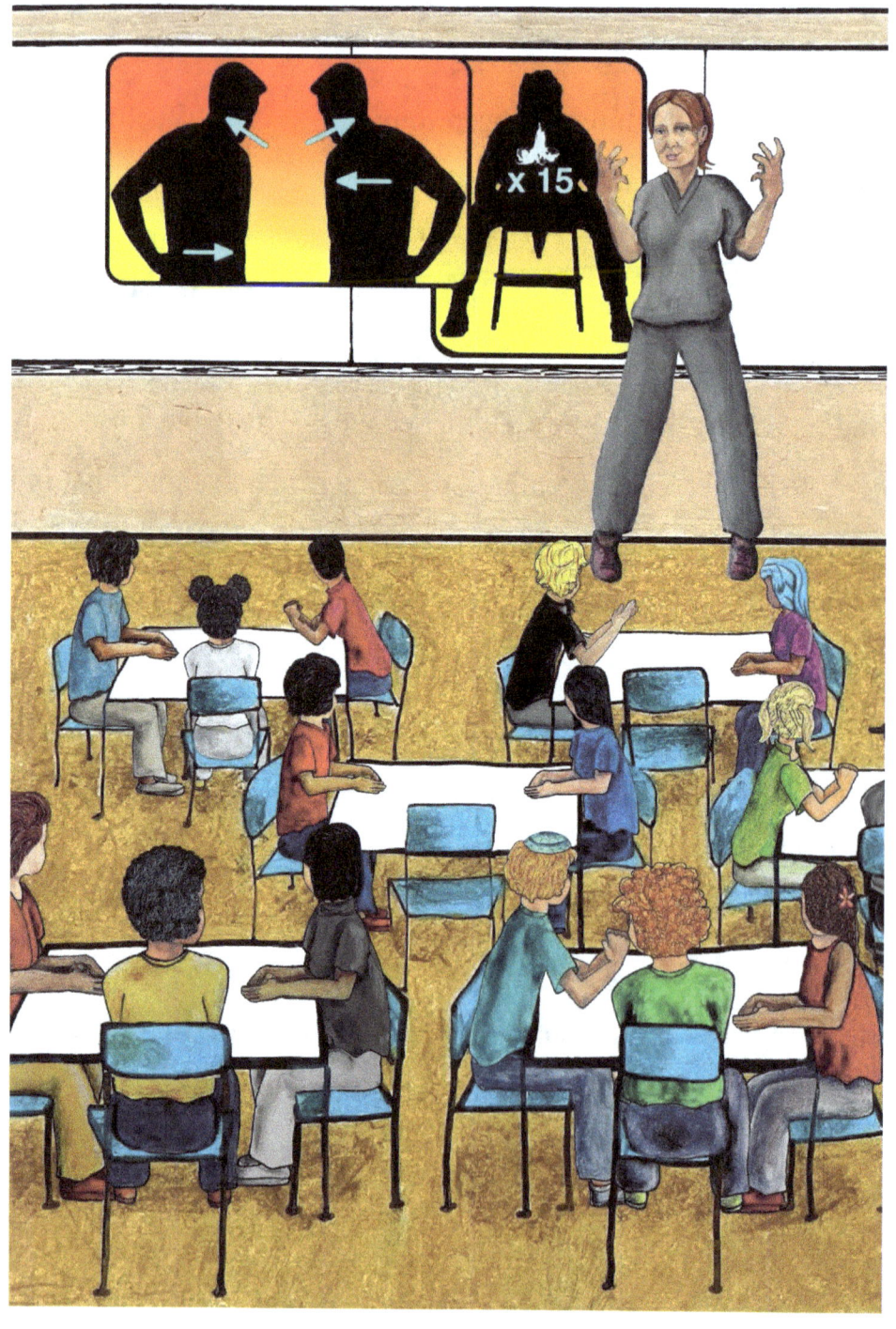

"Some have found that belly breathing instead of chest breathing can reduce anxiety. To practice this type of breathing, sit in a chair and lean forward by putting your elbows on your knees. Then, breathe for 15 breaths. I would like everyone in the class, those reading the book, and those watching the video to do this activity, so you can have another tool in your coping skill toolbox. Let's practice now."

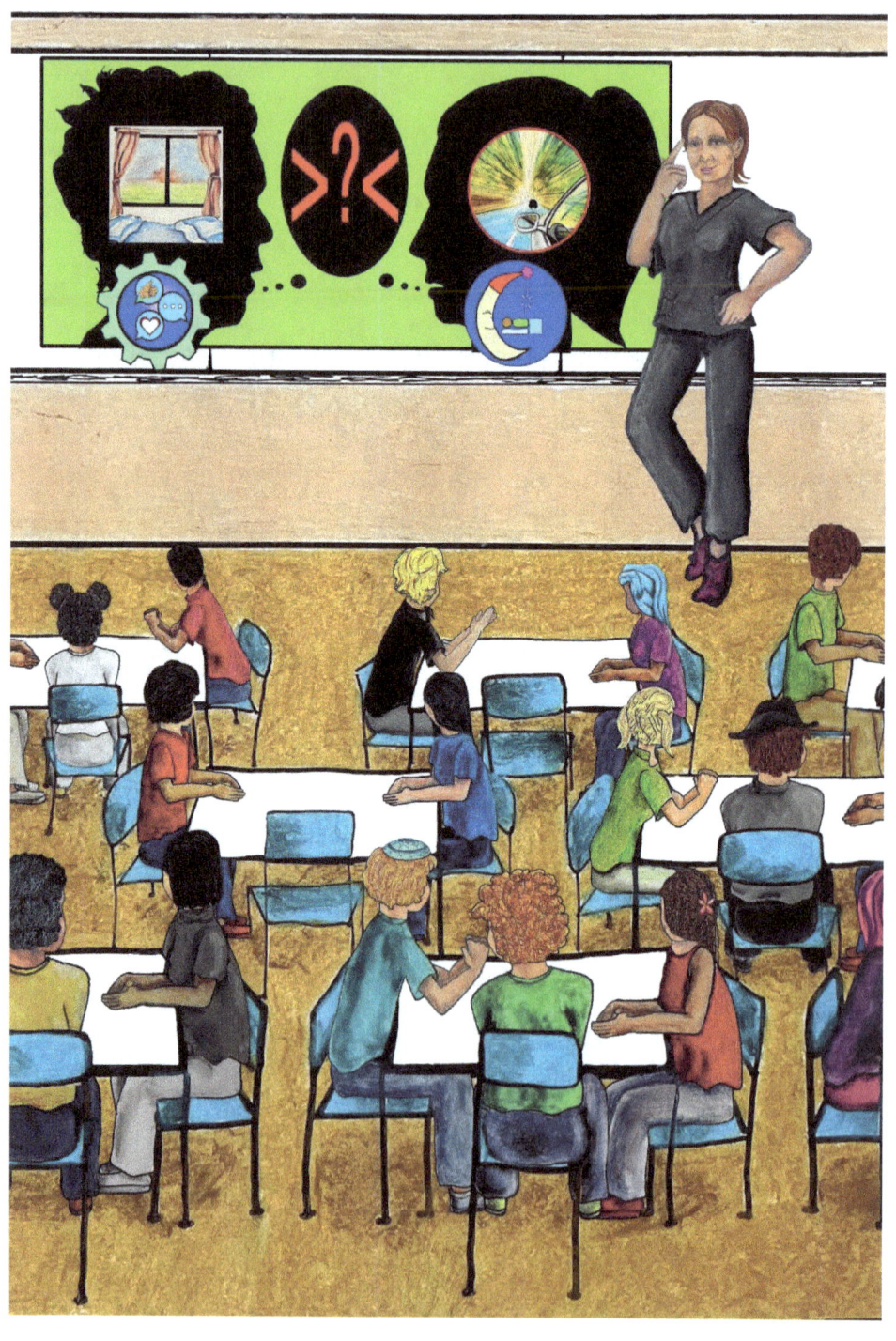

"Practice rituals of communication, since good communication can help with distraction, problem solving, and understanding other people. Always try talking to people in your vehicle about different things. Talk to your family members every night before bed. Use open-ended questions. A closed-ended question only requires the person to answer yes or no. Using the words 'tell me more' is a great open-ended question and encourages the other person to share many things about the topic that was discussed.

Schedule yourself downtime during the week and each day to not be overscheduled. If you live a life with constant demands from work and family, a person can live in constant anxiety, since they may feel there is never enough time to do everything properly. A person should manage their social media appropriately. You should develop good sleep hygiene, and get the proper amount of rest for your age and situation. If you are physically sick, then you will need a little more sleep than normal. It's a good idea to try to get extra sleep before a big event the next day."

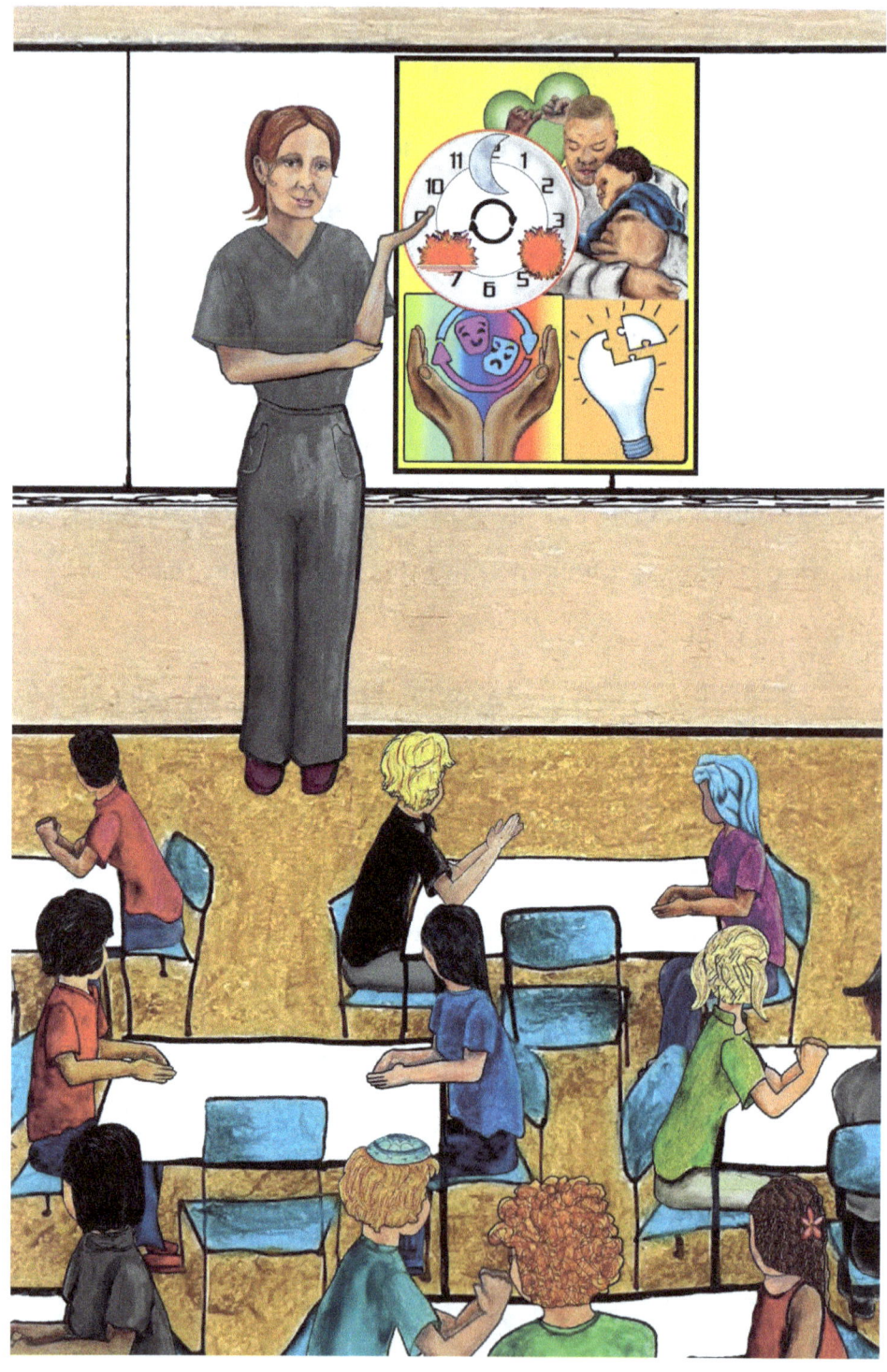

"We should all develop the skill of resilience. Resilience is defined by *Merriam-Webster* as the ability to recover from or adjust easily to misfortune or change. We will all experience change in our lives, so it is in our best interest to develop resilience. Changing perspectives is one technique that can help a person develop resilience. Having routines and keeping them can help a person develop resilience, such as exercising three times a week. Children having a safe and stable relationship with an adult is a great buffer for anxiety. If you are an adult, having a stable and healthy relationship with a mentor can be a buffer.

Having consistent daily routines is helpful, such as waking at the same time, eating around the same time, doing a favorite activity every day, and going to sleep at the same time. Connect with your peers, and have many friendships. Name your emotions, and try not to suppress them. Encourage yourself to problem-solve and help others solve problems, since that will help you get better at that skill. Practice self-soothing to calm yourself and exercise control when you can. Remember, going through difficult times will pass, and you will be on the next chapter in your life."

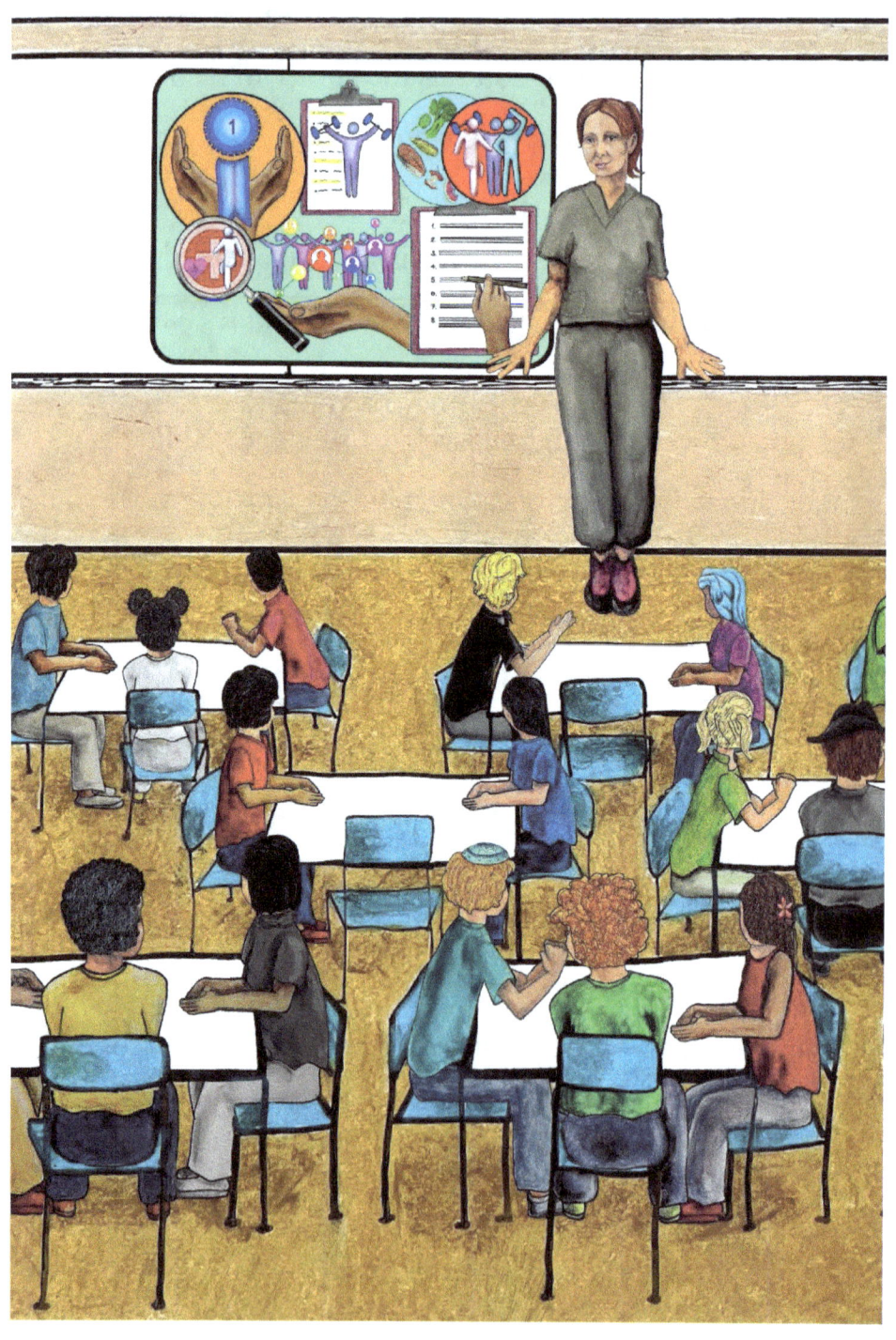

"Celebrate milestones. Not only your milestones, but also other people's milestones and achievements. Highlight your strengths as well as the strengths of others. Eat a balanced and healthy diet with lots of fruit and vegetables. Prioritize physical health and manage your medical diseases appropriately and with the advice of your treatment team. Exercise regularly by finding something fun that gets your heart rate elevated and causes you to sweat a little.

Maintain a good social support network and try not to burn bridges with anyone, since you never know when you might need them. Consider having a diary to write many different things down, such as your emotional states each day, triggering events, what your diet was, 3 good things that you experienced each day, and goals that were achieved."

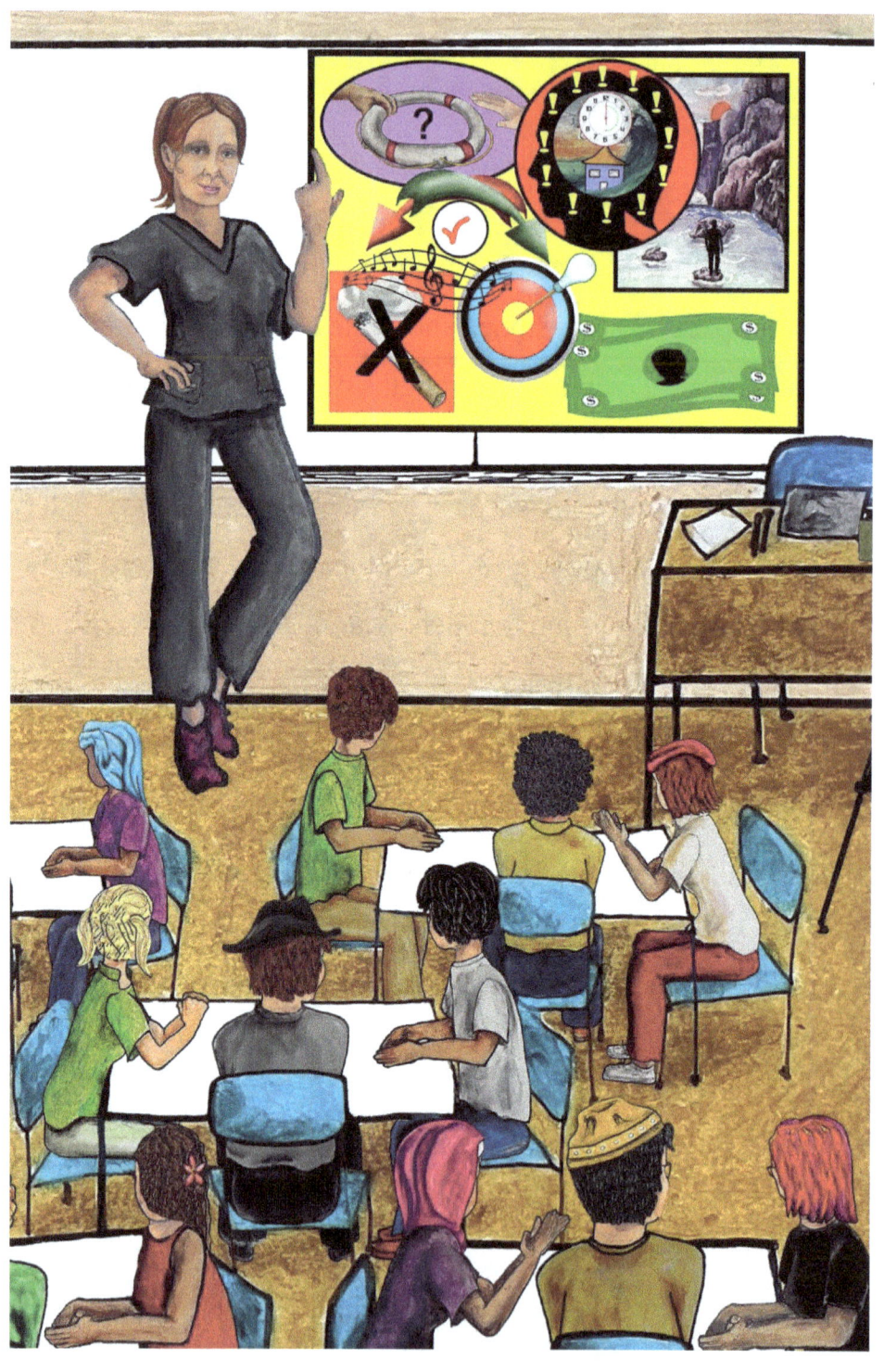

"Ask for help when you need it and even before you truly need it. Consider scheduling yourself to worry productively for 30 minutes each day. Focus on the problem and let the anxiety come about dealing with the event or situation, and then be finished worrying after 30 minutes. Think about your past choices to guide you to make even better choices. Practice music therapy since music has been found to help relax people and reduce anxiety. Go for nature walks, even if it is walking around a safe neighborhood for 30 minutes with someone else for safety.

Challenge your thoughts to see if they are valid when anxiety comes. Challenging yourself can be difficult, but the challenge is worth taking so that you improve yourself. If you have started smoking cigarettes, then get help quitting. Make smart daily goals that are specific, measurable, achievable, related to your overall mission and purpose, and time-oriented so that you have a deadline. Address your finances so that you have the resources you need to secure your necessities and achieve your dreams."

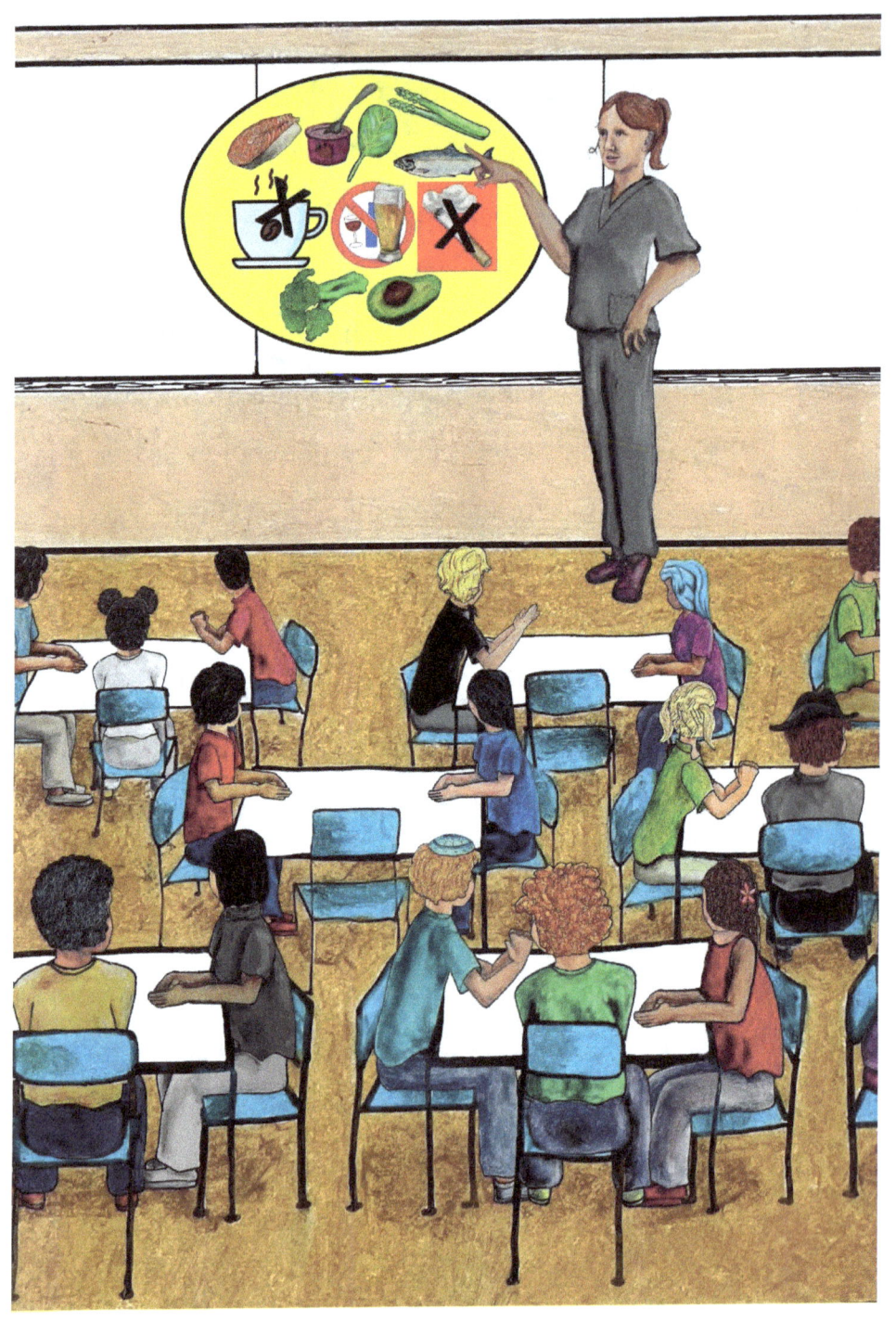

"For healthy eating, one of the best diets you can eat for your brain and heart is the Mediterranean Diet. Cut back on your sugar and processed foods, limit your caffeine, limit alcohol, and quit tobacco. Eat foods rich in zinc, such as whole grains, oysters, kale, broccoli, legumes, and nuts. Consume foods rich in magnesium, such as fish, avocados, and dark leafy greens. Eat foods rich in vitamin Bs such as asparagus, leafy greens, meat, and avocado. Try foods rich in omega-3 fatty acids, such as wild-caught salmon, and probiotic-rich foods, such as kefir, yogurt, and other fermented foods. Eating healthy gives your brain the tools it needs to work at its best."

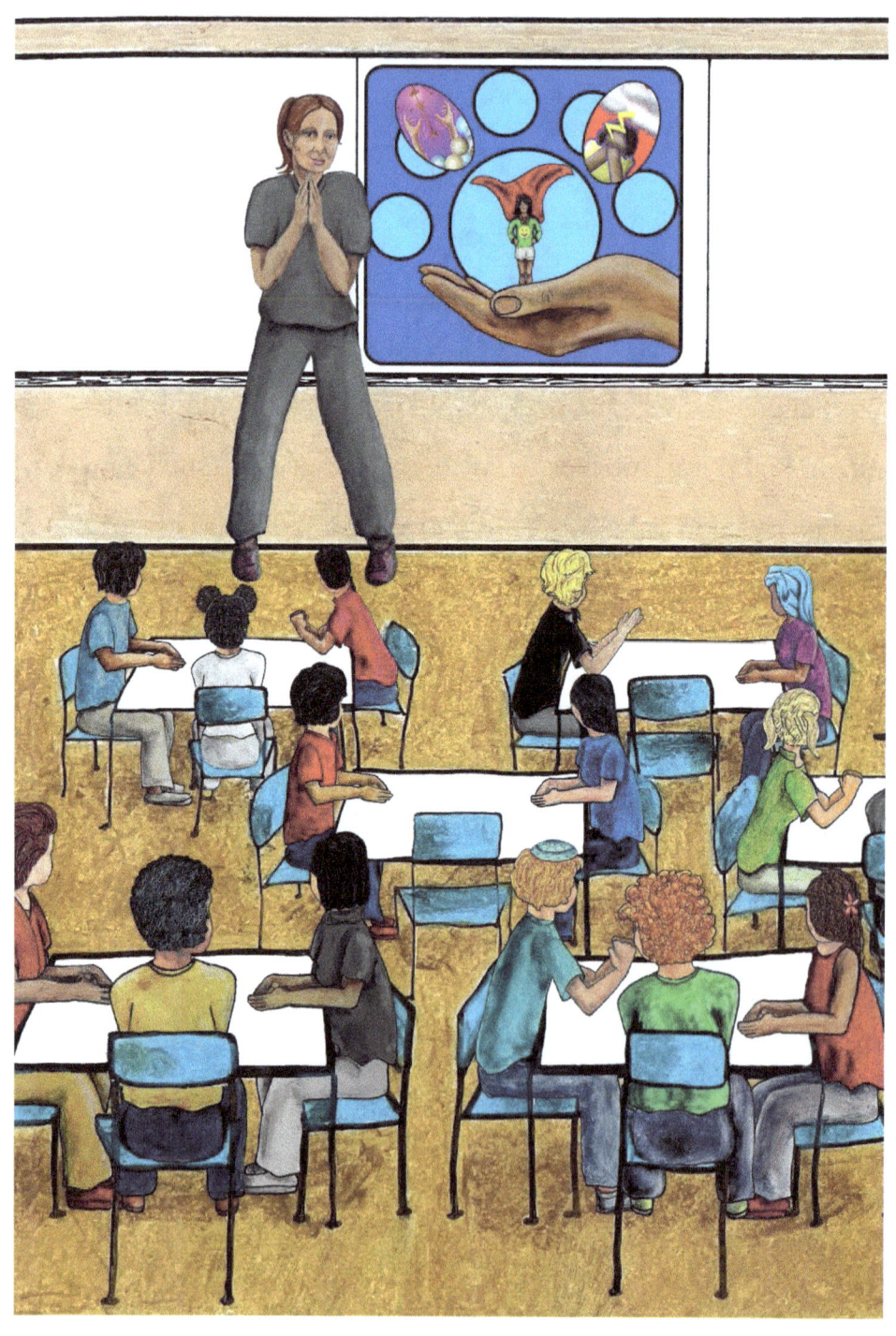

"Do your best to model confidence to those younger than you. Being a good role model will help future generations to better manage anxiety and stress. Allow yourself to have some level of distress. Preview anxiety situations with a young child in a safe place, so that you can allow anxiety to be produced but still be able to easily manage it with them. It's ok to try to narrate a young child's world so they have more words to explain what is happening to them. Expose a young child to a variety of situations so that they can manage their distress better.

Let them know that being an adult doesn't mean anxiety goes away or that it can always be easy to manage anxiety. Be willing to be vulnerable and open with young people, and let them know that it can still be difficult at times to manage anxiety or stressful situations. Life is a journey. Realizing that and appreciating the moment can help."

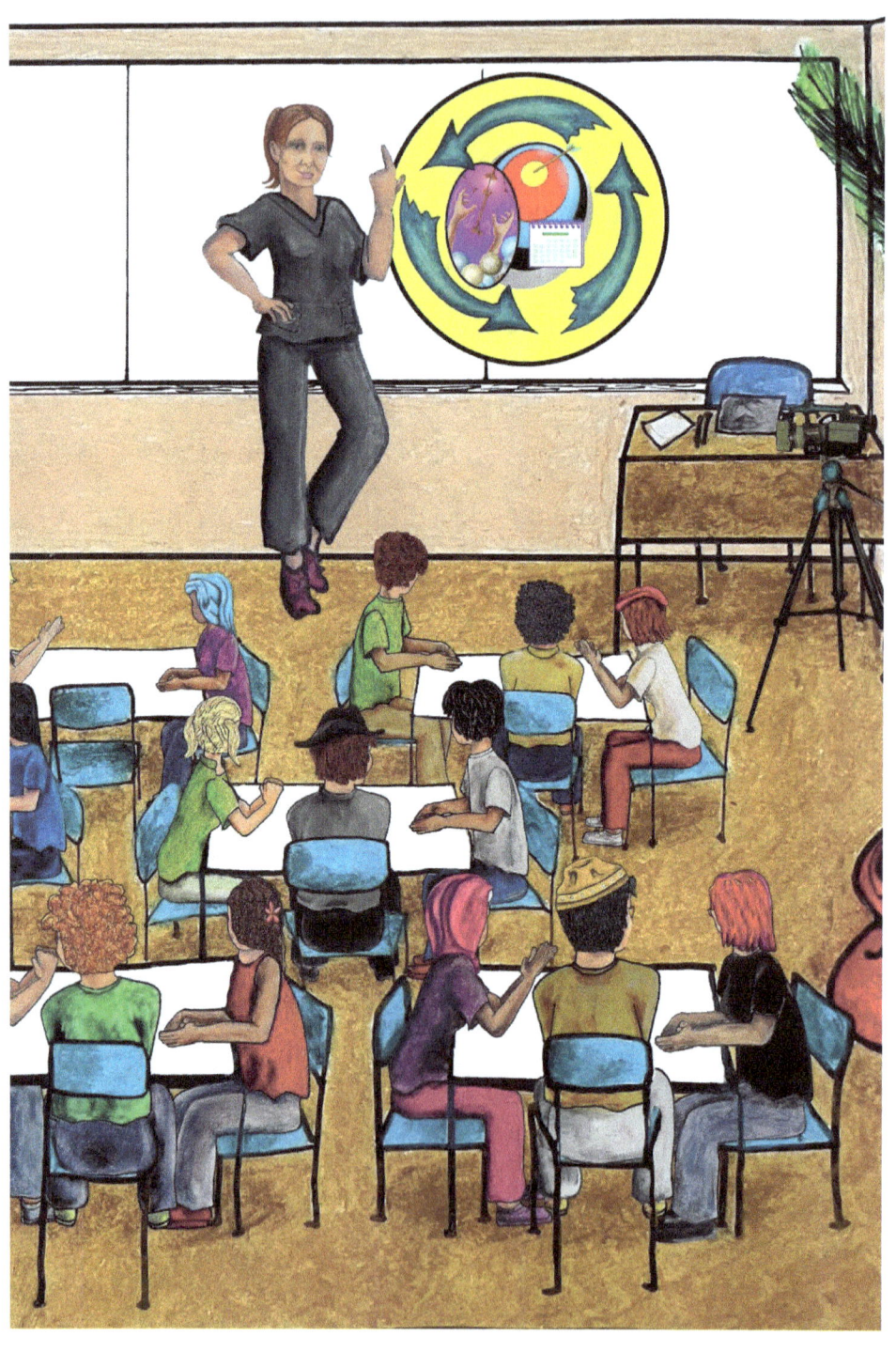

"Try to view anxiety as an adaptive response to our world. It can serve a purpose by showing a person where they need to take action about something. Try not to struggle with anxiety, but learn to manage your distress. Anxiety can be helpful for everyday life since it can help motivate us to improve our society. Avoid perfectionism since that can lead to a constant state of anxiety. Try using the idea of setting goals and prioritizing which goals will receive 100% of your effort and which others will receive average effort. Choose to be optimistic since sometimes it is a hard choice to make. The more optimistic you are, the easier it will be to find the bright side in a dark time."

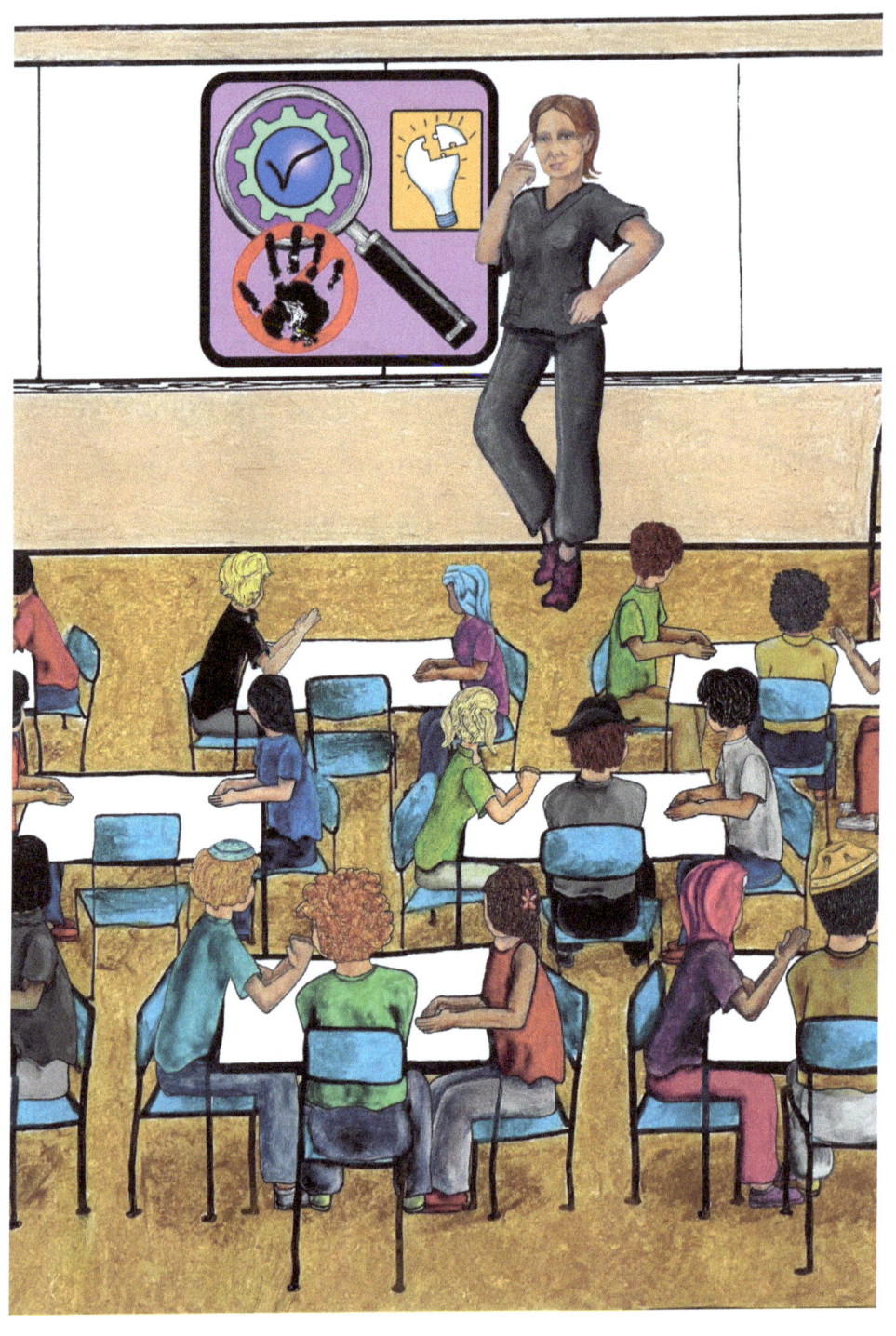

"Try assessing the situation as it is. You may need to distract yourself to help manage the anxiety, or it may be a situation where you may need to engage your problem-solving skills. Relax your body and reassure yourself that you can manage the situation. If you live with constant anxiety, get checked out by a psychiatrist. Ask for help when you need it.

We've gone over a lot of coping skills, techniques, therapies, and other points. Let's share with those around us a handful of strategies that we will try the next time we get anxious, since sometimes you must do many things to create a synergistic effect to drastically reduce anxiety. If the anxiety was produced by possibly many factors, then it may take many things to reduce it to a manageable level. Those of you watching the video or reading the book, think of some strategies that you will try the next time that you experience anxiety. Let's discuss these ideas with those around you now."

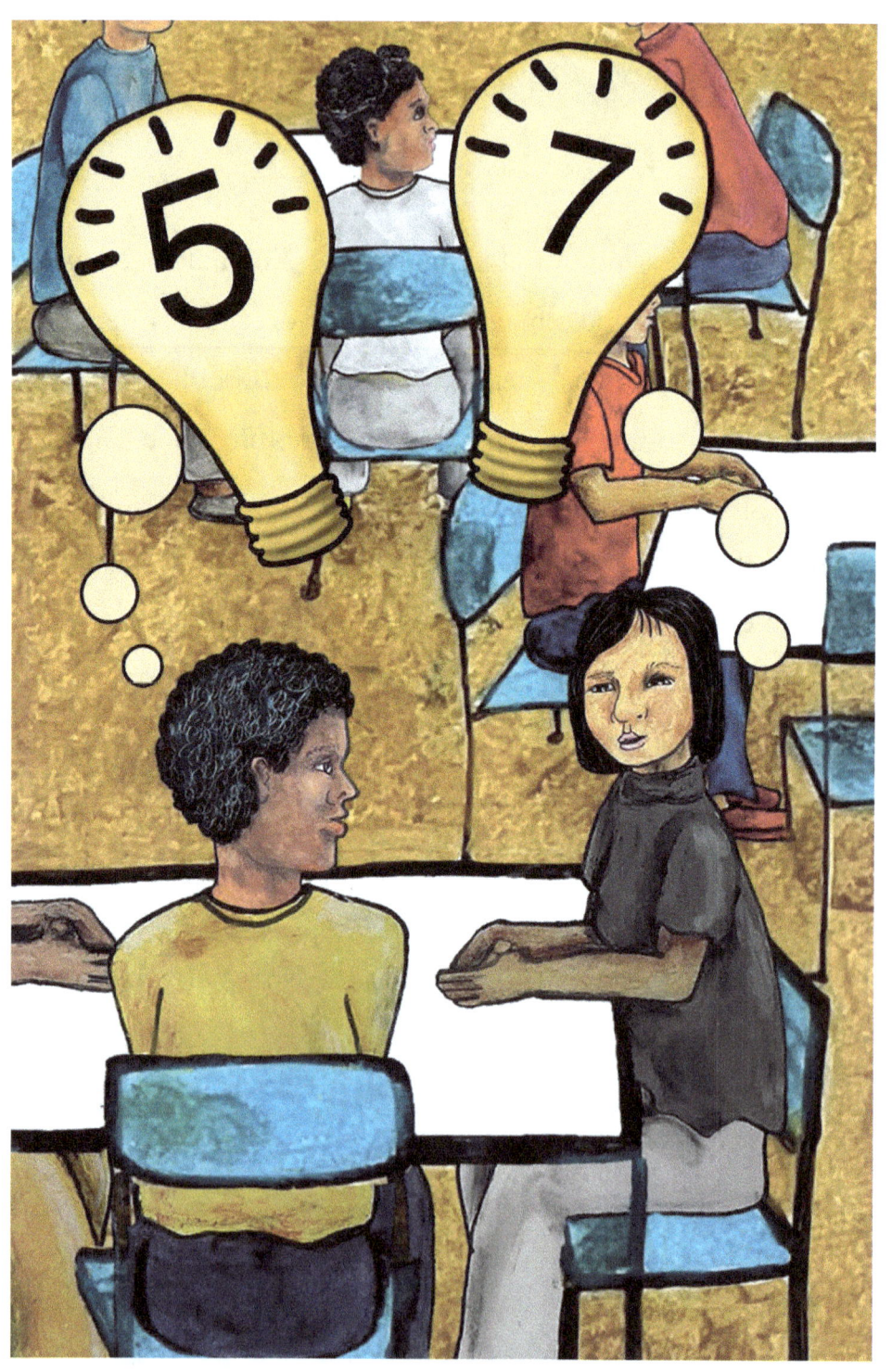

Ekon raises his hand, and Nurse Dorothea calls on him to speak. "I plan to deep breath first, then do perspective-taking to see if I'm missing something about the situation. I plan to start carrying a small bottle of lavender oil and will try aromatherapy. I will reach out to a friend and ask them if I am perceiving the situation appropriately. I will tell myself that I only have 5 minutes to be very anxious about the situation, and I must then develop some goals to resolve the situation in the best way possible."

"Very excellent ideas on self-soothing as well as reaching out to your support network," says Nurse Dorothea.

Lian raises her hand, and Nurse Dorothea calls on her to speak. "I plan to do some muscle relaxation and try belly breathing. Then, I will say a mantra repeatedly of 'you got this' for 5 minutes. I will identify the trigger and ask myself if it is rational to feel a lot of anxiety about the situation. I will try drinking chamomile tea if it is available, and highlight my strengths to myself. I will also start eating a more healthy and balanced diet with regular exercise and maintain a healthy relationship with my mentor to build my resilience capabilities."

"Very excellent to plan for long-term management through a healthy diet, exercise, and healthy relationships. Sometimes, you have to do future planning for future emotions," says Nurse Dorothea.

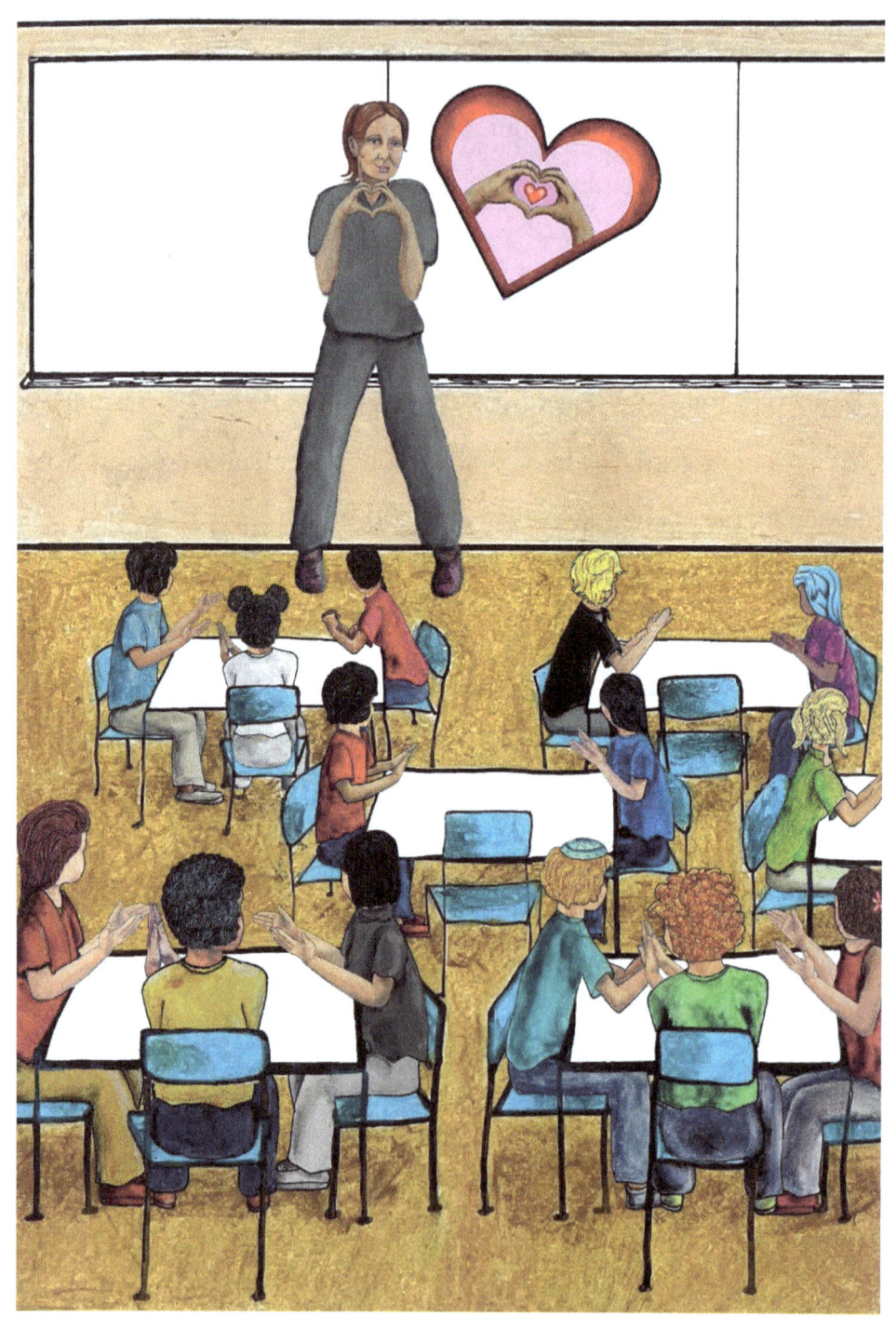

"I want to thank you for your time and attention to this mental health challenge. Anxiety can be viewed as a challenge for us to develop more skills and grow as a person. If we all develop greater knowledge, skills, and abilities as individuals, then we can increase our society's synergy to accomplish things that were once unattainable. We have much to do as a civilization, and we need to all do our part since we all seem to have a part to play in reaching our full potential. I hope you have a great rest of your day, and I'll see you the next time we meet," says Nurse Dorothea.

The class starts to clap, and some come up to the nurse and say 'Thank you, Nurse Dorothea' as they hug her.

References

Collier, S. (2020). What works best for treating depression and anxiety in dementia?
Retrieved from: https://www.health.harvard.edu/blog/what-works-best-for-treating-depression-and-
anxiety-in-dementia-202003182112

Collier, S. (2021). How can you manage anxiety during pregnancy? Retrieved from:
https://www.health.harvard.edu/blog/how-can-you-manage-anxiety-during-pregnancy-
202106252512

Collier, S. (2021). Postpartum anxiety is invisible, but common and treatable. Retrieved from:
https://www.health.harvard.edu/blog/postpartum-anxiety-an-invisible-disorder-that-can-affect-new-
mothers-202107302558

Coltrera, F. (2018). Anxiety in children. Retrieved from: https://www.health.harvard.edu/blog/anxiety-in-
children-2018081414532

Coltrera, F. (2018). Anxiety: What it is, what to do. Retrieved from:
https://www.health.harvard.edu/blog/anxiety-what-it-is-what-to-do-2018060113955

Corliss, J. (2022). Worry and anxiety linked to higher heart risk in men. Retrieved from:
https://www.health.harvard.edu/mens-health/worry-and-anxiety-linked-to-higher-heart-risk-in-men

Godman, H. (2023). A pill-free way to treat anxiety. Retrieved from: https://www.health.harvard.edu/mind-and-
mood/a-pill-free-way-to-treat-anxiety

Harvard Health Publishing. (2016). Managing worry in generalized anxiety disorder. Retrieved from:
https://www.health.harvard.edu/blog/managing-worry-in-generalized-anxiety-disorder-
201602179172

Harvard Health Publishing. (2017). Take steps to prevent or reverse stress-related health problems. Retrieved
from: https://www.health.harvard.edu/stress/take-steps-to-prevent-or-reverse-stress-related-health-
problems

Harvard Health Publishing. (2018). Trying to be perfect can cause anxiety. Retrieved from:
https://www.health.harvard.edu/mind-and-mood/trying-to-be-perfect-can-cause-anxiety

Harvard Health Publishing. (2020). Always worried about your health? You may be dealing with health anxiety
disorder. Retrieved from: https://www.health.harvard.edu/mind-and-mood/always-worried-about-
your-health-you-may-be-dealing-with-health-anxiety-disorder

Harvard Health Publishing. (2020). Overcoming anxiety. Retrieved from: https://www.health.harvard.edu/mind-and-mood/overcoming-anxiety

Harvard Health Publishing. (2020). Tips for beating anxiety to get a better night's sleep. Retrieved from: https://www.health.harvard.edu/mind-and-mood/tips-for-beating-anxiety-to-get-a-better-nights-sleep

Harvard Health Publishing. (2021). Focusing on past successes can help you make better decisions. Retrieved from: https://www.health.harvard.edu/mind-and-mood/focusing-on-past-successes-can-help-you-make-better-decisions

Harvard Health Publishing. (2021). Tuning in: How music may affect your heart. Retrieved from: https://www.health.harvard.edu/heart-health/tuning-in-how-music-may-affect-your-heart

Harvard Health Publishing. (2021). Pain, anxiety, and depression. Retrieved from: https://www.health.harvard.edu/mind-and-mood/pain-anxiety-and-depression

Harvard Health Publishing. (2021). Sour mood getting you down? Get back to nature. Retrieved from: https://www.health.harvard.edu/mind-and-mood/sour-mood-getting-you-down-get-back-to-nature

Harvard Health Publishing. (2023). Supplements for three common conditions. Retrieved from: https://www.health.harvard.edu/staying-healthy/supplements-for-three-common-conditions

Harvard Health Publishing. (2024). Recognizing and easing the physical symptoms of anxiety. Retrieved from: https://www.health.harvard.edu/mind-and-mood/recognizing-and-easing-the-physical-symptoms-of-anxiety

Harvard Health Publishing. (2025). Anxiety and stress weighing heavily at night? A new blanket might help. Retrieved from: https://www.health.harvard.edu/mind-and-mood/anxiety-and-stress-weighing-heavily-at-night-a-new-blanket-might-help

Harvard Health Publishing. (2025). Overcome your fear factor. Retrieved from: https://www.health.harvard.edu/mind-and-mood/overcome-your-fear-factor

Lee, E.H. (2022). Resilience: 5 ways to help children and teens learn it. Retrieved from: https://www.health.harvard.edu/blog/resilience-5-ways-to-help-children-and-teens-learn-it-202202242694

Marques, L. (2020). Do I have anxiety or worry: What's the difference? Retrieved from: https://www.health.harvard.edu/blog/do-i-have-anxiety-or-worry-whats-the-difference-2018072314303

McCarthy, C. (2022). The mental health crisis among children and teens: How parents can help. Retrieved from: https://www.health.harvard.edu/blog/the-mental-health-crisis-among-children-and-teens-how-

parents-can-help-202203082700

Naidoo, U. (2020). Eating well to help manage anxiety: Your questions answered. Retrieved from:

https://www.health.harvard.edu/blog/eating-well-to-help-manage-anxiety-your-questions-answered-

2018031413460

Nemours KidsHealth. (2023). Anxiety Disorders Factsheet (for Schools). Retrieved from:

https://kidshealth.org/en/parents/anxiety-factsheet.html

Salamon, M. (2023). Anxiety Overload. Retrieved from: https://www.health.harvard.edu/mind-and-

mood/anxiety-overload

Salamon, M. (2024). Co-regulation: Helping children and teens navigate big emotions. Retrieved from:

https://www.health.harvard.edu/blog/co-regulation-helping-children-and-teens-navigate-big-

emotions-202404033030

Salamon, M. (2024). Want a calmer brain? Try this. Retrieved from: https://www.health.harvard.edu/blog/want-

a-calmer-brain-try-this-202410293078

Solan. M. (2023). How to identify anxiety disorders. Retrieved from: https://www.health.harvard.edu/mind-and-

mood/how-to-identify-anxiety-disorders

Solan, M. (2025). Ease anxiety and stress: Take a (belly) breather. Retrieved from:

https://www.health.harvard.edu/blog/ease-anxiety-and-stress-take-a-belly-breather-201904261861

About the Illustrator

Lindsay acquired her BFA from Columbus College of Art and Design. She was a self-employed metal artist beginning in 1985 and was part of the American Arts and crafts movement of the late 80's and early 90's with an art piece on permanent collection at the White House and the governor's mansion in Ohio. The majority of the works she sold then were done in metal, either soldered or welded. During that time, she spent 5 years serving on the board of Ohio Designer Craftsmen and networked part of her business through them. She sold many of her works through art galleries across the USA and Japan. She did many individual commissions and was also commissioned to do giftware design through Bath and Body Works, i.e., the Limited, in the year 2000.

In 2008, Lindsay went back to college to acquire another degree so she could try her hand at teaching high school art. She acquired a M.Ed. from U of A. She taught art at 6 different schools in AZ before retiring in 2022. In her last 4 years, she taught: Art 1, Advanced Art, AP Art, Ceramics, Advanced Ceramics, and Photography I, II, III, and IV (which was also producing the school's yearbook). Several of her students were recipients of HAA Art scholarships. During her first year of teaching at public schools, she taught Graphic Design. All this time, she enjoyed making art with her students and building her illustration, drawing, and painting skills.

During those teaching years she still accomplished a few commissions of steel sculptures. It started with the first commission from Norton Abrasives of creating the company's mascot. It was a larger-than-life French bulldog named Cooper. Cooper resides at the company's US headquarters in Brownsville TX. The mascot had long lines during one trade show of people wanting to take selfies with it. It was a hit and resulted in a personal commission for a couple in Los Angeles of another bulldog named Sebastian.

When Lindsay retired in 2022, she worked with an old friend in Ohio who is an author and performer on a children's book. All the illustrations in the book including the cover were created by Lindsay. The book is for 0-8 year old children and is called "Sleep Little Raven".

Lindsay has kept a blog since 2008 showing the progress of her works at www.curlycu.com.

In Lindsay's words:

"Making art is like breathing; it is a must for my own survival and sanity."

About the Author

Michael is married to Perla in Tucson, AZ. Michael served in the US Air Force between 2002 and 2010 as an Electronic Warfare Officer on the EC-130H Compass Call and deployed 6 times in the Global War on Terror. Michael then served 8 years as an Army Wounded Warrior Advocate. Michael used his GI bill to go to nursing school and works as an RN at an inpatient psychiatric hospital in Tucson, AZ. Michael enjoys listening to Beethoven and reading a lot of news.

Michael's college education:

B.A. in Psychology from Auburn University,

B.S. in Biology from the University of Alabama at Birmingham,

M.S. in Management from Troy University,

Master in Health Administration from the University of Phoenix,

M.S. from the University of Arizona through the accelerated Master's Entry to the Profession of Nursing program

Other Books by Dow Creative Enterprises®

For more information about the series, visit

www.NurseDorothea.com

Visit www.DowCreativeEnterprises.com for more

information

www.ingramcontent.com/pod-product-compliance
Lightning Source LLC
Chambersburg PA
CBHW060458260626
47161CB00005B/2164